1

I was driving to a long-awaited physical therapy evaluation, pulled into the parking lot, and suddenly I no longer had control over my right leg. It jerked when I was trying to press the gas pedal. It was a huge office complex, but I could not find the place I was supposed to go, so I had to keep circling in the parking lot. I was unable to see the words clearly on the little signs at the entrances to what seemed like a hundred businesses. The car jerked along with my leg. I had lost all control of my leg and foot. I finally found the office, with both feet on the brake, parked in the handicap spot, and tried to regroup.

There were some strange sensations moving through my right calf and foot, but I couldn't have begun to describe them. Armed with my four-pronged cane, I was determined to get to my appointment. I scooted along, using my car and the cane to get to the sidewalk in front of my handicap parking spot. From there, I used the front bumper to propel myself as far across the sidewalk as I could toward the brick wall on the other side.

The office was only about 30 feet from where I was, but I needed a plan because there were plants in a mulched area between me and the door. I was trembling and off balance. My right leg and foot would not do what I asked them to do. I had to figure out how to negotiate the part of the wall I could reach, and see if that momentum could help me past the landscaping to get to the door. Since I had stopped, I had no momentum to work with yet. What's worse, it ran slightly uphill.

Dragging one leg at a time and using the cane to push myself forward, I inched toward the door. Sometimes I moved sideways, using the cane for whatever leverage I could get. It was August in Florida and ridiculously hot. I was soaked with sweat and in tears off and on along the way. When I got to the door, I realized I couldn't open it because I had nothing to brace my legs and body against for leverage to pull. I tried, but it did not budge. I wasn't sure I wasn't going to pass out right there. The windows were tinted, but I could see inside. I wondered if anyone inside could see me standing there, yet unable to open the door. Tears were welling up. It wasn't like me to be this late for anything. Someone inside finally saw me there, and came to open the door.

I was more than 30 minutes late, which was how long it took me traverse the 30 feet from my car. I apologized for my tardiness and hoped the physical therapist could still see me. He did.

I was still trying to use my cane, which was an exercise in futility not lost on the physical therapist who evaluated me. He said I needed to lose the cane, get a walker and perhaps a wheelchair, and that I needed in-home physical therapy because I should not be driving a car.

In my defense, or maybe my stubbornness, I desperately shared with him that my walking and driving hadn't been great before, but that this deterioration just happened, explaining what went wrong when I pulled into the parking lot. I remember thinking if I had not had that appointment, I could have been driving home from work in rush hour traffic when my leg failed me. That notion sent a ripple of panic through me, so I tried to focus on his evaluation.

As part of it, he asked me to use my feet and toes to make letters. I swore I would have been able to do that when I got up that morning, but I could not move my feet at all to make any part of a letter. I tried to use my whole leg to do it, but he said that was cheating and he needed to see if I could use my feet. This was crazy, I thought, of course I could do it. So I picked the letter "I" and tried harder. Nothing. I decided I could not be trying hard enough. I was not sure how to feel about it. I felt a level of frustration unlike anything I had ever experienced.

What in the hell was happening? Would it come back again later and was this just a fluke—some fleeting symptom like some of the others I had been having? Surely, it was not really this bad. Sitting there while he evaluated me was torture. My mind was racing and I was trying every which way to convince my feet to do what they were asked. I tried to make my feet move, but nothing happened. He was asking me to do things I did not know I could not do. I did not understand. I was confused by my body's betrayal. I was breaking a sweat again. I thought this had to be some kind of mistake, so I would try even harder to do his little exercises. I could not.

It was rare that I could not will something to happen in my life when I wanted it badly enough. Well, it was rare until my illness first showed itself six months earlier. Since then, I had begrudgingly learned to surrender to my symptoms one by one, and that exerting my will against them was futile. My head was spinning. I thought I might pass out or throw up before the evaluation was over. I kept shaking my head, trying to deny the surreal, cruel reality of my failing limbs.

This lack of control over my body was unlike anything I had ever experienced, and I was at a loss what to do about it. I just continued along with the evaluation and figured I would deal with getting home when it was over. All I could do was go moment to moment. The therapist seemed annoyed about the doctors who had referred me for outpatient physical therapy. I was actually trying to defend them and appear to be not as bad off as I seemed. I did not want him writing anything in my record that said I was not allowed to drive or something.

Clearly, I should not be driving, but I would get home before making that decision myself. My defensiveness was the only coping strategy I could muster. I did not want to break down or throw up like I felt like doing because I did not need another professional writing in my medical record that I was "overly emotional" or having some sort of "conversion reaction." As a psychotherapist myself, however, I have to say that having a meltdown right there in the parking lot after I pulled in, would not have been horribly inappropriate.

    I had gotten myself into that physical therapy office with just the cane and it was pretty obvious that I would need more than that to get back to the car. The physical therapist walked me out to my car trying to let me use a walker, but I wanted to show him how I got there with the cane. The entire way, I was saying, "See, I can do this." I was using the building wall, the cane and his body for support for the first bit to show him how I got into the building. I tried the walker for the remaining 20 feet or so. Using the cane and him for support did not work well at all. I could not push off him to propel myself forward. The walker really did not help either. How did I ever make it from the car to the building? The poor guy had to have been shaking his head at me insisting I could do it when he and I both knew that I had no control over my feet. He likely had more awareness of my denial than I did.

    Still in denial, or perhaps delusional, I dismissed the difficulty I had getting back to the car. I got there, so there was no sense belaboring the entire nightmare. I thought that maybe when I got to the car things wouldn't be as terrifying as they were when I arrived. I was thinking that maybe I had overreacted, as if the past two hours had not really been so bad. Once I got in and started the engine, I tested myself and found that my right leg and foot were still jerking when I tried to press on the gas.

    My left foot seemed to work on the brake, but the brake was not going to get me home. I was taught that you use the right foot for braking and on the gas. If I concentrated, I could remember to use my left foot to brake, and I had been using both to brake for a couple of months already. I wondered if I could somehow use my left foot on the gas pedal too. Still in my parking spot and out of gear, I tried that idea, but ended up revving the engine without any sense of control. I decided it would not be wise to try that on the road. So, as frightening as it was, I decided my safest option was just to use my unruly right foot and leg.

    I prayed harder than I had ever prayed. I prayed I did not have an accident and hurt someone. I prayed to keep breathing and not freak out while I drove. I could freak out once I got home. I just needed my leg and foot to cooperate for about five miles. I bargained with God that if I did make it home safely I would never drive again. It was late morning and traffic was light.

My Hyundai Santa Fe was an automatic, but the way I was making it lurch and stutter it must have looked like someone driving a stick shift and doing a lousy job. The car jerked as suddenly and unpredictably as my leg. I was trying to press on the gas smoothly but my leg was shaking my foot right off the pedal. I would have to lift my leg with one of my arms to get my foot back on the pedal. I had to keep doing that to keep moving forward.

I would take some deep breaths to try to relax my leg, but it did not help. My insides were churning. I tried driving slow and even put on my hazard lights. I would press hard on the gas pedal, my foot would jerk off it, and I would coast until I got my foot back onto the pedal. I considered pulling off the road and trying to call someone to come get me, but everyone I knew was at work and I just didn't want to bother them anymore than I already had. I was determined to get myself home.

At stoplights -- and in Florida the lights seem to take five minutes -- I would try to regroup and relax the death grip I had on the steering wheel. The tears would start, but I would fight them off. This was no time for a meltdown—not yet. My neck and shoulders were stiff from the tension; my jaws were locked in a clench that would not release.

At last, and after what seemed like hours, I was just a couple blocks from my house. I was going to make it. My heart was a jackhammer when I pulled into the driveway and turned off the key. I somehow opened the door and pulled myself to my feet. I locked the car door, and stood uneasily for a moment, thanking God I did not kill someone.

Once in the house, I wanted to scream and cry or throw up. I wanted to call someone, but could not imagine how I would describe what I had just experienced. I would cry and then make myself stop crying because I needed to focus, to try to figure out what to do next. No one was there to help me do that. I couldn't pace back and forth on my feet, so I did my pacing in my mind.

My brain was a pinball machine, and my body was staging a coup de ta. I chain smoked and tried to focus on giving my dogs some attention. They did not like it when I cried, so I would tear up, stop, tear up, and stop. They licked the tears from my cheeks.

2

The first time I saw them they were huddled together in the back corner of a cage at an animal shelter in my Ceredo-Kenova, West Virginia. They were brothers, black lab mixes, maybe eight weeks old. I was told they were huddled that same way when they were found next to a country road after their mother had been hit and killed by a car. I made eye contact with the smaller of the two and he began to get to his feet and inch his way toward me. About half way, he turned to look at his brother, who then also started toward the front of the cage. Before I knew it, I was holding them in my arms, promising them they would never have to be in a place like this again.

I fell in love and adopted them on that hot July day in 2001. I named the smaller of the two, Duke, and then my roommate named the other Amore'. That was nine months before they would hop in the backseat of my Toyota Tercel for a road trip with me to Florida. Soon our new home would be a two-bedroom house with a fenced-in yard in Safety Harbor, a quaint little town nestled on the west shore of Tampa Bay.

I had no inkling then that these two sweet-faced kiss dispensers would become my sentinels, motivators and greatest source of strength in a fight I could never have imagined coming. The closeness we shared and the commitment I made to keep them together are cemented in my heart. My bond with my boys--that is what I called them--is central to understanding how I managed to get through my nightmare or even be here to tell about it.

My parking lot drama and breathless drive home that

fittingly ended with my boys lapping up my tears, struck me as a good a place to begin my story. Though it happened six months after my symptoms first showed themselves, it was the day the harsh reality of my illness grabbed me and shook me. After that, it was harder to be in denial, harder not to accept that I would soon be in a wheelchair.

Using a wheelchair to get around was not part of my plan when I left Huntington, WV, in early March 2002.

My motivation for making the 1,000-mile trek south was my need to put far behind me the heartache of a failed marriage, followed by a failed four-year relationship. Since I was going to move anyway, it made sense to go where I would be close to family. Both my father and brother and their families had been in Florida for years.

Nevertheless, for me, starting over was going to be considerably more difficult than making a geographic change and getting over failed relationships. Along with my luggage, the familiar darkness of my lifelong struggle with depression came along as it always does. It has followed me like my shadow since childhood, a malady I have countered with medication and therapy with varying measures of success.

Although I wondered how anyone could be depressed for long in a state where the sun always seems to shine, its soothing warmth was no match for the dark clouds that stalked me. Within nine months, whatever benefits the sun had first provided me had worn off. I slipped into the same depressive and fearful state I had been trying so hard to escape. The only real differences were that I had a new address where I was a part of my family's life, and I was increasingly dependent on my dogs for my strength. I decided I would resume antidepressants, find a psychotherapist, and start in a less obsessive way to work on my issues.

I could not have known that my depression issues soon would be driven to the breaking point by a mysterious motor neuron disease, one that would present me with the most terrifying challenge of my life.

By the time my calendar had flipped to July, I had been in

Florida six months and had managed to create much the same life I had left in West Virginia. I worked as a therapist with the homeless, taught adjunct introductory psychology courses at a local college and joined a basketball officiating association. Most of my time was spent working, so any social network I might have had was limited to coworkers or family. I was never good at developing social support, so when my symptoms started eight months later in March of 2003, I had only a few people I considered friends. It was really just my dogs and me.

My disease did not attack in a single bound; rather it crept up on me, at first just showing itself in bits and pieces. I would sometimes have trouble separating the coffee filters or gripping a water bottle lid to open it. One day, I was fixing my mailbox and my right arm gave out on me, suddenly zapped of its strength. The strange and intermittent collapse of the muscles in my arms and hands had been going on for about a month when I found myself losing my balance and landing on my face at the dog park. I conveniently convinced myself that Duke was somehow tripping me, perhaps bumping me as he played or ran alongside.

Since the symptoms were so varied and seemingly unrelated, I didn't see a doctor right away. Instead, I kept thinking I would wake up and it would all be gone. But it did not go away, so after about a month of denying it, I scheduled my first doctor's appointment. By then, whatever was wrong had put me behind on my case notes at work because I couldn't press down hard enough with the pen to write. I was beginning to use walls and parked cars to help get me get from one place to another.

I also had no idea that my first doctor's appointment would be the beginning of an exhausting and futile parade of specialist visits and hospital stays with the same result: no one could pinpoint exactly what was wrong with me.

The depth of my feelings of powerlessness, lack of control and despair was evident to others in my world as the disease took hold in the early months. Its progression became as rapid as it was cruel, each day finding me worse than the day before. I fought my legs, my arms, my hands and my feet as they found new ways to confound me. I somehow managed to walk and drive far longer than I should have. Some of that was stubbornness; the rest of it misguided determination. I expended a great deal of energy resisting and fighting my body.

    I vacillated from feeling defeated and wanting to crawl into a hole, to knowing that I was not done yet in this life and needed to keep trying to move forward to see what might be on the other side of this struggle. But moving forward has a completely new meaning when you cannot get your feet to go where you want them to or propel yourself forward with your own legs.

    Getting out of bed and getting to the bathroom was not only difficult, but also dangerous. I could not open my own jars and bottles, or make my bed. I did get a shower seat at Walgreen's one day on my way home from work, but could not even open the box by myself, so a coworker came to help me. Showering became a bit safer after that. It was exhausting to bathe and put on clothes. Fixing food was never my forté, but that became significantly less important since I usually didn't have the energy to eat. I was still going to work, although I was drained before I got out the door.

3

It had been about four months since my symptoms began and whatever was wrong with me was exacting a heavy toll in every aspect of my life. My deterioration was as obvious to my therapy clients at Directions for Mental Health as it was to my students at St. Petersburg College. I had used up all my sick leave, found a roommate to assist me and help me stay in the home I rented and where I wanted so desperately to stay with my dogs. I had lost my ability to walk without leaning on things to keep me going forward. I could no longer do the simple, everyday things. My body was fighting me relentlessly.

When I tried to walk, it felt like cinder blocks were tied to my legs and my feet were encased in cement. I could propel myself forward if I pushed off a wall, but when I did that, I knew there was a chance I might lose my balance and fall face first. My legs were stiff, my feet were already contorting any way they could to try to move me forward, and my joints ached.

The best leverage I could muster came from the back right side of my right heel. I had at least a shred of stability there. It enabled me to sort of drag my left leg up to meet my right one. But that maneuver really only worked if I was leaning against something. There was no part of putting one foot in front of the other that came easy, and the amount of energy it took to try was enormous.

At home, I relied heavily on the walls in my hallways. There were only a couple of spots where there were no walls near enough to help me get from room to room. I fell a lot, but after the first few times, I learned that I could get to where I was going faster by being on the floor and sliding across the tiles. So I began orchestrating my own falls. I would push myself off a wall, drop to the floor, and keep moving forward in a kind of wounded soldier crawl. There was a certain forward momentum generated by the fall that would almost make the first part effortless. Mostly, I was going from the bedroom, down the hallway, and out the patio doors to watch Duke and Amore' in the yard. I also went out there to smoke my Marlboro Lights.

    I was getting pretty good at navigating my own environment, but involuntary falls were becoming more frequent, and I was concerned about hitting my head. If I knocked myself out, who would know besides my dogs, and I honestly didn't want to freak them out any more than I already had with my rapid decline. I also knew that if I sprained or broke something, what little mobility I had would be seriously jeopardized. Safety was beginning to outweigh my own stubbornness and resistance to assistive equipment like a walker or even a wheelchair.

    It was early July and my college summer class was ending. My mounting symptoms had become an obvious source of concern for my students. They had watched me get worse with each passing week and some of them often walked along with me to make sure I made it safely to my car.

    I told them I was interested in getting a roommate and to let me know if they heard of anyone looking to share a place. I was missing so much work that I needed help with my rent. The only way I knew for sure that I could keep the dogs and I together was to keep the house. I also was becoming increasingly fearful of living alone, and knew I would be safer with a roommate.

    Within a couple of weeks, I had one. She was a young veterinarian technician and student who had a little white ankle-biter dog. Although she was only with me a couple months, her timing could not have been better. Her love of animals was a bonus. She was there when Amore' had his first grand mal seizure--

a treatable convulsive fit not uncommon in dogs--although we weren't sure that was what was happening at the time.

And she was in the house with my boys while I was hospitalized at Tampa General Hospital three separate times in August. I was there for a week each time, undergoing painful spinal taps and an endless array of tests. It was the scariest time of my life, and my fears were compounded by still having no idea what was wrong.

My third hospital stay began the day after my terrifying drive home from the physical therapy evaluation, the day I promised God I would never drive again if I got home safely. That afternoon, after I thought I was all cried out, I left a phone message with my doctor's nurse, a message that must have been hard to understand because I started choking back tears again as soon as I began speak.

But my tearful message got through and I got a call back that evening from the doctor who had overseen my tests during my first two hospital stays. She persuaded me to be admitted again for yet another spinal tap – lumbar puncture in medical parlance – and another round of tests. She tried to reassure me, telling me that this time there would be a new group of specialist trying to finally unravel the mystery of what was happening to me.

That third hospital stay also ended without a definitive diagnosis, although they were at least able to rule out some possible causes including multiple sclerosis. So the frustrating and terrifying quest for a diagnosis would continue while my life was falling apart.

But one positive arose amid the intrusion and pain of that third hospital stay. I confronted and was able to overcome my dread of wheelchairs, and once I got in one, I concluded that having one would not be so bad after all.

Although I was placed on fall precautions when I was admitted, no one offered me a wheelchair. I decided to ask for one because it was taking far too long for a nurse or an aide to come to my room to help me get from the bed to the bathroom and back. I do not remember exactly what the one they brought me looked like. Just standard hospital issue, I guess, brown plastic seat and back rest, lots of stainless steel. I felt conflicted when I first sat in it. How could it have come to this already? While I didn't exactly embrace the idea of having one, I quickly began to enjoy the freedom of movement it provided. In the back of my mind, I hoped having a wheelchair would improve my attendance record at work and allow me to continue doing what I love.

The next thing I knew, I was wheeling up and down the hospital hallways. On flat, smooth surfaces, I could make my arms wheel me along pretty well. I could get myself to the bathroom far faster and safer in the wheelchair than clunking along with a walker. It was almost liberating. It had been months since I could do anything quickly.

However, there was nothing quick about my wheelchair smoke breaks. The smoking area was a long way from my room and there were lots of hilly sidewalks and curbs along the route. I could not quite get my arms to wheel me up the inclines, nor could I control my speed going down. When I did succeed in getting to the smoking area, I could not get back without help. I was at the mercy of a random nurse also out for a smoke or an aide who would have enough sympathy to join me, and then help push me back and open all the heavy doors we encountered.

Just the same, this wheelchair business was not the horrible thing I had conjured. I couldn't remember anymore why I thought being in one would be abhorrent. I used to think that people in wheelchairs could not walk at all. I am not sure where I got that idea, but it was one of the reasons I convinced myself I did not need one. A wheelchair also represented giving up or giving into my new reality. It meant, in my mind at least, I might never get out of it. I was still going to bed each night with the expectation of waking up back to my old normal self.

I knew I no longer had the energy to use the walker and that using one was not that safe. The wheelchair just made sense. It was a safer, more energy efficient tool for getting around and I decided I would use one from that point forward. I count that, along with my decision to stop driving, as two things about which I exercised some freedom of choice. I had no idea that those two choices would be among the easier ones I would make as time passed.

    I also could not have predicted then that a wheelchair would be my ride through a nightmare in which I would lose everything before a flicker of light helped show me the way out.

4

He was my in-home physical therapist. He showed up at my house a few days after I got out of the hospital that third time, and he was there to evaluate me and to do a safety evaluation of my home. After he determined the level of my mobility, he surveyed my place for safety issues so that he could order whatever assistive equipment I would need. The only thing on my must-have list was a wheelchair since they did not give me one when I left the hospital.

His name was Greg, a tall guy with kind eyes. He was easygoing and compassionate but he wasn't letting me get away with anything either.

I tried to convince him that I could hobble around, so he asked me to show him. I showed him and he cringed. He tried to get me to use the walker with him guiding my steps, but he almost lost me when I started to fall. My feet were not flat on the floor anymore, but contracted sideways with the outer sides the only thing really touching the floor.

I thought I could do it better with shoes on, but I found out the soles of my shoes had taken on the same contorted shape as my feet. I could only hobble, forcing my twisted feet to propel me forward any way I could. It was not pretty. The only way I could move forward with the walker was to press down on the handles, lift my legs, and swing them forward like a gymnast on a pommel horse.

He decided we should do it a different way. I knew this was his way of saying that it was not safe to practice trying to walk right now and that was okay. Instead, he wanted me to try what seemed to me like simple exercises. One of them involved lying on my bed with my back propped against the pillows and trying to bend my feet at the ankles back toward my head. When I tried, nothing happened, but he insisted I keep trying anyway. It seemed futile to me and frustrating, so I challenged him, asking what was the point in trying if I could not do it.

He told me about some research that proved the brain is more likely to tap into muscle memory, and something about needing both hemispheres of the brain to make the action more likely or coherent. I am science-minded and tend to listen if research is cited, so I agreed to keep trying. This time I strained hard enough to break a sweat but still my feet did not budge. I began to cry and asked him if this was really necessary. I then became angry with him. I thought he was lazy because he was not helping me do anything and I saw no point continuing.

However, he was persistent, citing more research about the brain recognizing the movement I am imagining, even if I was not actually able to do it. I just shook my head, silently vowing to fact check him later, and kept trying.

Even though my feet didn't move, the idea was to send the signal through my brain and my body as if they were. Through the duration of our eight sessions together, I could never make my feet move on that exercise.

My dogs were excited to see company and nearly bowled Greg over when he arrived for each session. We tried closing my bedroom door while I was doing my exercises, but Duke insisted on coming in to make sure I was ok. Duke lay on the bed beside me and Mo eventually would lay down in the floor of the spare bedroom just outside the door after barking and pawing at the bedroom door at first. It helped me to have Duke there beside me during the sessions. Doing something I clearly could not do was a lot easier to swallow when I had my hand on one of my dogs.

My boys were just as curious as me two days later when a big white durable medical equipment van pulled up in front of the house and this guy made his way up my driveway with the special equipment the physical therapist had ordered. I remember being pleasantly surprised with what he brought.

    Besides a manual wheelchair, which was really all I expected, my delivery included an elevated potty chair, and a much steadier walker than the one I had. Although I had never understood the purpose of the elevated potty chair with arms, boy oh boy, did it ever make my life safer in the bathroom. Before I got it, I had been using the small countertop around the sink to hoist myself on and off the toilet, but since my legs had become so uncooperative, I had pretty much just been letting myself drop and landing hard on my butt on the seat. I could not seem to control how quickly or smoothly my legs would let me sit down. At our next session, I thanked Greg for knowing I needed that.

    But more than anything, it was the wheelchair that kept me hopeful. Having it meant I could return to work, and work seemed to be the only normal thing I had anymore. I was great at being a workaholic and was born to be a psychotherapist and more than ever before, I needed the distraction of someone else's problems, and I needed to be needed. I had been struggling with feeling useless, and work surely would help with that, or so I thought.

    My first day back to work in the wheelchair was a Monday, and I wheeled myself in behind my desk about 8 am. It was pretty uneventful until I had to use the staff bathroom about two hours later. I went to a regular stall, and then realized that I had to get from my chair to the toilet seat. It took me a few minutes, but I was able to do it safely. The drama started when I was finished and found I could not get up. There I was, pants down, sitting on the toilet, unable to hoist myself up. The staff bathroom had two stalls, so I would have to wait until someone came in who could help me. Meanwhile, I tried to make my legs raise me up. They could not. I tried to figure out a way to get leverage, but the toilet paper holder and other things attached to the stall were too unstable for me to pull or push on. As I sat there half-naked, I began to wonder if anyone even used that bathroom regularly. My thoughts were racing and so was my heart.

    I did not know the routine of my new coworkers since this was my first day there in my new position. I started to work myself into a panic. What if no one comes in at all? My last resort would be to try to drop myself to the floor and maybe I could do my wounded soldier crawl out the bathroom door. But how would I open the door? I would not be able to get myself back into the chair once I landed on the floor from the toilet seat, so that would be something I would try only as a last resort. If I could not get off the toilet, what made me think I could get up off the floor? And if no one came in, would anyone even know to look for me?

I have no idea how much time had passed when someone finally walked in, and I told her my predicament. I had only met her a few times when I was doing homeless outreach therapy, and this was my first day as her colleague in the day treatment program. She may have been all of five feet tall and was petite. She lifted me up from the toilet, helped me to pull up my panties and pants, and get me over to the wheelchair. I worked on trying to button my button-fly khaki's once I was back in the chair.

I would never wear these pants again because buttoning button-fly pants sitting down with a tremor was ridiculous. I was shaking, my hand tremor was worse and it was taking forever to button my pants. We stayed in the bathroom for a bit while I tried to compose myself. I was trembling and tears streamed down my face, but I was trying to keep it together. I had clients on the other side of that door, so now was not the time for a full out breakdown.

My rescuer's name was Cara, who was a case manager who and worked down the hall from me. She was awesome and acted as if it was just another day at the office. She kept asking me if I was okay and then asked how long I had been stuck in there. I had not been there very long, or at least I did not think so.

I remember being glad I wasn't in a single stall bathroom where you lock the door when you enter. I had not taken my cell phone in there with me. One part of me was crying and shaking because I was imagining how it could have played out. The other part of me was crying and shaking because someone I hardly knew had to lift my naked ass off the toilet and help me pull up my panties. I was grateful, tearful and mortified by the experience on so many levels. It was not my first lesson in humility, nor would it be my last.

Apparently, I needed an elevated potty chair there too. I had no idea I could no longer get up from the toilet. That was a particularly mortifying way to learn about something else I could no longer do.

The bathroom where I was stuck was in an older part of the building. It did not have a handicap stall, though there were plans to change that. The client bathroom did have a handicap stall, but the clients were schizophrenics and chronically mentally ill folks who had some strange bathroom habits. My alternative was to go upstairs to use the newer bathrooms while they tried to make the downstairs bathroom more accessible for me.

I did not go to the bathroom the rest of the day. In fact, I tried not to go to any part of the building where there weren't other people around, and if I had to, I took my cell phone. I had no idea what I might need anymore. What else could I not do? Could I not do anything by myself? I was the epitome of needy and vulnerable, which were two things I tried desperately not to be all of my life.

The bathroom incident was further evidence of how everything in my life had gone awry in the seven months since my symptoms began. I had lost much of my independence and my career working with the homeless had taken a detour.

The new day treatment therapist position was my third job with Directions for Mental Health in six months. While it did not include me working directly with the homeless, which had always been my passion, I was blessed and thankful that I was still working at all. I was able to stay there only because my employers were flexible with me and allowed me to set a schedule and caseload I could handle. I was really fortunate to have such great bosses who advocated for me to stay on even after I had exhausted my Family and Medical Leave hours.

Nevertheless, I missed working in the field and meeting with the homeless where they were—at the beach, at the soup kitchen, wherever. I first began working with the homeless in West Virginia, and was immediately struck by their humanity. They were no different from me. Many were professionals who once had successful careers. They became broke and homeless when one set of circumstances would be compounded by another set of circumstances.

I loved learning what those circumstances were. I loved advocating for them with social service agencies to get them what they were entitled to, from food stamps to medical care. I developed relationships with all of the agencies so that my clients could get what they needed and in many cases, I could get them off the streets and into shelters. I got many of my clients into one shelter program in particular, the Homeless Emergency Project (HEP) in Clearwater. It was the place where my clients who were unable to work would go, and where I would see them for ongoing therapy and case management.

Although I was still working with the homeless in my new job, my clientele were mostly chronically mentally ill and substance abusers. I still did some individual therapy, but most of my time was spent doing group therapy. It would not have been my first choice, but at least it was a job in the field I loved, and for all I knew my last hope for making enough money to keep my dogs and me together.

But deep down I was terrified I was going to end up losing my dogs and even become homeless myself.

5

My father's name is Bob Swain. He spent decades in the financial business where he had, and at 70 still has, a strong work ethic, a trait I apparently came by honestly. He is soft-spoken and there is warmth in his brown eyes behind his black-rimmed glasses. I would not describe our relationship as warm and cuddly, but there has always been a closeness between us, a kind of quiet devotion to each other, like the way it is between many fathers and daughters.

He is the one who drove me and my wheelchair to work that first day and for as long as it would take my paperwork to clear the way for me to start being driven to and from work by a wheelchair transport service. As it turned out, dad's tenure as my ride to work lasted close to two months because my original paperwork got lost in the shuffle, never got to my doctor for her signature, and I had to apply all over again.

I liked my morning rides with dad, who always brought breakfast of some kind and coffee, just the way I like it, two creams and extra sweeteners. I was not sleeping well and tended to be overly chatty in the mornings. My dad just is not the chatty type, though sometimes our conversations escalated into uncomfortable conflict. One sore spot was money, since he was trying to help me to get my finances in some sort of order. But the touchiest subject was my dogs. He was always trying to convince me they were too much for me to handle, and that I should find them a new home. I know he had my safety at heart, but he just did not understand the bond I had with my boys and that not having them in my life was never even a consideration for me.

While disagreement traveled with us from time to time, our morning rides began to foster growth in our relationship and the way we communicated. I wish I could have protected him from everything that was going on with me, but I also needed his help and understanding too much to shut him out. Most of my life, I would just withdraw whenever I was struggling, never wanting anyone to see the struggle or feel obligated to do anything to help, which especially went for my dad.

But he has always been there for me when I allowed him to be, which before this disease struck, had not been very often. And something I didn't find out until much later was that for much of the time he drove me to work he was suffering from Shingles, a viral condition that causes a painful rash. And he didn't just drive me. He lifted my wheelchair in and out of his van and pushed me up the long ramp to the office door. He never complained, not a whimper.

In addition, throughout the same period my dad got me to work, I got a ride home from my boss, Dan Herper, who lived south of our offices in Clearwater, not far from my place. He did so with the blessing of his boss who agreed to let him take me home whenever I was ready, which often was after only a few hours because I was just too tired and weak to continue. They may not have been my family but my employers treated me as if they were.

I wasn't chatty on the way home like I was in the mornings with dad. I was exhausted and often feeling down, a mood Dan quickly sensed and countered with words of encouragement. One of the most validating people I have ever met, he knew I was not the broken, scared, out-of-control person I feared I was becoming, and often reminded me of my own personal power.

I appreciated his attempts to lift my spirits, but it was hard for me to shake the ambivalence I felt about going home at all. I dreaded the reality that awaited me there, the aloneness with my own thoughts spiraling out of control I guess, and a sense of the walls closing in on me.

At least there was comfort in knowing my boys would be there waiting for me, their unconditional love taking away a little of the sting of getting home to be alone with my fears. They greeted me with kisses and then clung to the sides of my wheelchair as I rolled myself through the house. I would eventually get settled on the bed and they would be up there with me, pawing at me to pet them before sharing space together on the bed. While home was always my refuge, in those days it was only Duke and Amore' who made it that way.

My dogs aside, getting home from work was no longer the welcome down time it was before I got sick, a time that suddenly seemed so long ago. Instead, it was when the fears and uncertainty that came with this damn disease tried to engulf me. It was when my head filled with disturbing what-ifs. What if I wake up even worse tomorrow? What happens if I can no longer pay my rent? What will I do if I lose my dogs? What if I cannot work? What if I fall and hurt myself? What if no one can tell me what is wrong? What if no one can fix this? One chain of questions created another, and another, until there was only overpowering fear.

The initial burst of enthusiasm about the wheelchair and getting back to work had waned dramatically in the first couple of months, and work had done little to bolster the sense of personal power that Dan so often reminded me I had. Being trapped in the bathroom that first day turned out to be a harbinger of how being at work would become progressively difficult. I had counted on work to be my refuge from the rest of my reality, but in short order, work had become its own harsh reality with no place to hide.

My first wheelchair issue at work was not being able to open doors from my new-seated position. Turns out, you have far less leverage sitting down than standing up, which lets you put all your weight on your planted feet so you can pull a door open. My center of gravity had changed, my arms were weak and every door in the place was much heavier than I remembered – never mind that I was sitting on wheels that rolled. I had no idea how to navigate in a wheelchair outside of my house and hospital corridors. I also had no idea that I did not know how, and I had never considered asking for guidance in that area from my physical therapist. After all, a wheelchair is pretty much self-explanatory, isn't it? You sit in it and roll the wheels with your hands. How hard can it be? I never considered that the simple act of opening a door would be any different sitting down. I also needed to be pushed up the ramp outside because it was long and my arms simply weren't strong enough to do it.

Our program included serving lunch for the clients, so during this time, everyone was in the main area. I could never get through that area because of chairs and clients who were not great at paying attention to passersby.

My physical limitations were compounded by the stress I felt from all the attention I was getting from coworkers. They meant well, I know, but their endless inquiries about my health overwhelmed me.

It had been several months since many staff members had seen me and they had no idea how rapidly I had deteriorated. Each time I encountered someone I had not seen for a while, I would have to explain. I did not have explanations. I still had no name for what I had. I tried hard not to talk about any of it while I was at work, so sometimes I barely answered them. If I did not talk about it, then I would not have to worry about having a total meltdown when the reality hit me.

That absolutely could not happen at work and so far had not happened anywhere. I am not quite sure how it had not happened, but I was expending a lot of energy preventing it. I was afraid if I broke down, I might not recover. It may have been the only thing over which I seemed to have some control. Work was supposed to be my escape from my nightmare. It was where I could pretend I was ok, even though I was far from it and everyone knew it, including my clients.

So there I was, my ever-worsening condition making me dread going to work when I already dreaded going home. It was with that mental state as a backdrop that I was about to get a terrifying, prolonged lesson in just how vulnerable I had become, and it came courtesy of someone you would think I could trust implicitly: my wheelchair transport driver.

Once I was approved for wheelchair transport -- technically called Demand Response Transportation or DART -- I was assigned the same driver to and from work nearly every day. I still lived in Safety Harbor, so I was going from home to work in Clearwater, and then from work to home with the same driver.

Over the course several months, I probably got too comfortable with him. On the way home from work, when I was exhausted and vulnerable, I probably shared way too much with him. He would often challenge me to get out more than just working. I would tell him work was challenging enough, but that didn't seem to faze him. He finally talked me into going out to eat with him. I did not realize until a few weeks afterward that he was actually hitting on me. I thought he was just being nice.

He often seemed harsh when he was trying to convince me to do things I simply did not have the energy to do, but since I was so overly sensitive about everything then, I thought sometimes he had valid points. I did not realize until looking back on it later that his approach was to bully me into hooking up with him. He often said things like how much easier it would be to have a man around to keep me company and to do things for me. I was not at all interested in him romantically and for the longest time, I just thought he was trying to get me to stop thinking in terms of limitations. Perhaps on some level he was, but he did have an ulterior motive.

That became frighteningly clear one day when he was raising the van's wheelchair lift with me on it and began bullying me into going out with him. I angrily blurted out a pretty rigid boundary for him, making it clear that he and I were never going to happen. I did this as he was raising me in my wheelchair into the air on the lift to get into the van. As I saw his reaction, I knew it was an untimely mistake.

The driver controls the lift. Your chair is on a piece of metal that is controlled electronically. If you are not all the way up or all the way down, you can't go anywhere. You are suspended. Once you are in the van, the driver straps all four wheels of the chair to the floor of the van. He stopped the lift, looked at me with anger boiling in his eyes and said, "You won't have much of a choice since I am the one controlling this lift."

"Excuse me?" I snapped back at him. "Lower this lift, I will call and get another ride home from a different driver."

"What?" he said. "You think you can call and report me? No one is going to believe you. I am the golden boy of all the drivers. Besides, you cannot get another driver tonight. You are at my mercy."

I was exhausted and was not going to continue to engage him in this drama, but I also had absolutely no way of getting out of the situation either. I had experienced various degrees of vulnerability since my illness began, but at that moment I was the most vulnerable I had been in my life. I was on the lift, suspended in the air. I could not get out of my chair or off the lift even if I had needed to, so I was, just as he had said, entirely at his mercy. That realization sent chills through me and I needed to try to use the only thing I had to help me—my brain. I changed my approach to one of quiet resignation.

I let him think he had worn me down, even though I was scrambling my brain trying to come up with some way to defend myself should it escalate. I essentially apologized to him for upsetting him, acted as if I was the one in the wrong and hoped that approach would work. My tactic seemed to calm him down.

My heart was still racing. I felt like I would shake out of my skin, but was able to appear calm. He said he was not serious about his threats and wanted to be friends. I simply said, "Please just take me home, I am really tired."

It was too late in the day when I got home to call his supervisor. The same driver drove me to work without incident the next morning. I called from work soon as I got there and sensed immediately that he was right about his supervisors not believing me. I doubted a report was even filed. Regardless, I was assured that that driver would never be assigned to transport me again. That had to be good enough, even though it was not. What about the next unsuspecting girl in a wheelchair? I simply did not have the energy to wage an all-out war over it.

I was assigned a new driver effective that afternoon. It took a while to get a regular driver, and in the interim, I spent a lot of time waiting for late drivers. I never knew if that was by design. Anyway, it never happened again with another driver.

If being vulnerable had become a way of life for me, I vowed never to allow a sense of helplessness overtake me. It would take more than a driver with bad intentions to keep me from figuring out how to better handle all of this. I could have launched an investigation and raised all kinds of a stink about what he did, but also knew that the fight in front of me would require all my energy.

6

After about six months, I had had it with the limitations of my manual wheelchair, its little spinning, squeaky front wheels and its two bicycle-tire size back wheels that were sometimes impossible for me to push. I had put off efforts to get a power chair far too long, clinging to the false hope I was either going to get better or figure out a better way to get up and down ramps and sidewalk curbing. I finally put my misguided logic aside and tried to get a power chair.

I should have known that getting one wouldn't be easy, either. My insurance company kept denying my doctor's orders to approve me for one, claiming it was not medically necessary. While I waited out the insurance denials, a coworker who had come to my house to build a ramp for my front door offered to let me borrow a family friend's power chair that wasn't being used.

It was red with a black vinyl seat on it and it reclined. It was designed for someone much bigger than me, but I made it work anyway. It was nice to be able to zoom myself around work and to be able to duck out and hide from people for a breather if I needed it.

Eager to expand my newfound freedom away from work as well, I embarked on a trip to a popular mall in Clearwater to both get a haircut and try out my new wheels in a busy, public setting.

I wore my hair short back then and it was a good thing I did because washing and rinsing it had become a chore. The shorter it was, the easier it was to take care of since my arms were so weak. I had found a hairdresser I liked at the same mall when I first moved to Florida, and found out she worked Sundays and sporadically through the week. Wheelchair transport did not run on Sundays, which I found out the hard way when I planned to go the first time on a Sunday. I finally coordinated with her for a different day, and scheduled my first mall excursion aboard my loaner power wheelchair.

  What I noticed first was that wheelchair transport drops people off and picks them up at only one spot at the mall. This spot at the mall has no automatic push button door, nor is there a sidewalk that leads you to other entrances at the mall from the parking lot. I found this a bit disturbing and was so glad I was not in the manual chair for this adventure. Since I could not open the door into the store where I was dropped, I decided to wheel through the parking lot to get to the nearest entrance with an automatic door. The cars driving in this area of the parking lot were merciful and I made it to the next entrance without incident. The haircut and eyebrow waxing-- my first of anything done with my eyebrows in nearly six months because of my hand tremor-- went off without so much as a hitch. Off I went to the few stores I actually like to visit at the mall before my transport home would be there.

  My first store was right beside the hair place. I liked to look through the sales racks there. The sales racks are in the middle of the main aisles of the store. I did not realize that walking people could not see me because I was below their eye level and suddenly people were nearly falling into my lap as they rounded a rack of clothes. There was no real way to get out of the way. I was becoming startled by people coming unpredictably from behind the clothes racks. I couldn't see them, they couldn't see me. Whatever illness I had also gave me an exaggerated startle reflex, which would start my legs jerking.

  I gave up on the sales racks and went in search of a new bra. In the lingerie part of the store, the aisles were very small. If it was not on the outer edges of the area where the lingerie was, then I was dragging bras and panties off the racks with the arms of my chair to the floor. I dragged some bras and panties and realized I was going to make a mess if I continued to shop here, so I decided I would just try a different store. The aisles were far too narrow for a wheelchair, and this power wheelchair was wider than most.

My favorite Hallmark store had moved a few storefronts up from where it used to be. I had to figure out how to get there. I had always taken the steps and had to find the ramp to take me there. I was okay with going farther into the mall, had time before wheelchair transport was to pick me up and after all, I was autonomous, right? The Hallmark store seemed so much smaller than I remembered.

I went in a couple of the aisles where there were no other people, but then became fearful of "break it, buy it" store signs. I decided to leave the store before I accidentally broke something that I did not particularly want to buy. Still feeling optimistic about this newfound autonomy, I was sure I could shop somewhere. I could go anywhere I wanted now that no one had to push me. I headed for another store I used to like, and immediately wondered if they had added more aisles to make them all smaller? There was no way I was getting through there without knocking merchandise off the shelves.

Thirsty and a bit disappointed in this adventure, I went to the food court. First, I had to find the elusive elevators. They are hidden around the back of the mall's centerpiece ice skating rink, and I don't believe I had ever used it. I had to look at the signs and the mall map to find it. Nearly run over by people who didn't see me down here and feeling as if I had to dodge quickly moving ambulatory people, I decided to just stop at the closest vender. It was the cookie store and they had the diet coke I wanted. The counter at the cookie place was so high that even if I had been standing up, it would have been high. I ordered a chocolate chip cookie and my diet coke and tossed my money up onto the counter best I could. I could not reach the straws or napkins up there, but could see them. I asked for help to get those when the girl working tossed back my change. I couldn't really reach my change and she didn't help me get a straw. Maybe she couldn't hear me all the way down there? I stopped at another vendor with regular counters and took one of their straws.

It had not been the autonomous, independent trip that I had in mind. I did not realize I would face so many obstacles wheeling through the mall versus walking through the mall. I was certain of one thing from the experience--I was glad I had never really enjoyed mall shopping anyway. Otherwise, I might have been even more disappointed. I counted the haircut as the outing's only success.

I was getting the message: autonomy and independence had become relative concepts, if not illusory. Precious little in my world now did not require help from someone. I wondered when I might settle into this realization, break down the walls I had always kept around me and allow those who wanted to help me come inside.

For now, my sense of being alone and disconnected intensified with each new loss I incurred, from the onset of another frightening symptom to finding another everyday thing I could no longer do. It seemed that whenever I thought things could not get any worse, they did.

I had spent most of my life in as much isolation as I could create. While I always had people in my life and was always there for my friends and family, I was never able to let down my guard enough to let others into my inner world. I had few close friends because to me, being vulnerable and needy was equated with certain death. Yes, I had been taught at an early age that you couldn't count on others to help you and that you could only count on yourself. Somehow, I translated that lesson into it being life threatening to need someone or to appear vulnerable.

Ironically, just three months before my symptoms began I had concluded that my issues with never wanting to be vulnerable had been limiting me. I had been actively working on it with my therapist and those closest to me, an effort stopped short when my body failed me. My inner world was dark and the darkness was the filter through which I viewed the world outside of me. There were periods of light, and the light was nice until I fell into the darkness once again.

Feeling lost and alone

Unable to move
Unable to hide
From proof of my reality.

Feeling scared and trapped
Unable to run
Unable to hide
From the darkness of my truth.

Feeling angry and sad
Unable to cry
Unable to hide
From the loss of what was my life
2/29/2004--THSC

    Still in denial of the permanence of my situation, I seemed to believe that if I could just ignore these bizarre symptoms, they would go away. I still went to bed every night with the genuine expectation that I would wake up and find it had all been a bad dream. Each morning, as I began to notice something else on my body that was not working right, I would lose a bit of that part-denial, part-optimism that it would just all pass. I was young and relatively healthy, so as the symptoms continued to show themselves, I became increasingly frightened about keeping my home, my dogs, my jobs and my money.
    It was a notion that turned prophetic.

7

    The calendar had flipped to March 2004, which made it one year since my symptoms began and my life as it used to be, my life with an everything-works body, the life I took for granted, ended. It was an anniversary that would not be marked by a celebration, but rather by all that I had lost and a crushing fear that I may never get better.

I had not been able to drive for six months. I could not stand safely and was in a wheelchair. I was working fewer hours, having trouble keeping up with even the simplest of daily living activities, and still the doctors were unable to determine what I had. I had already lost my adjunct teaching position and had been shuffled around to different positions where I worked. My car was repossessed on Dec. 7, which was also my 33rd birthday.

My income reduced to a trickle and desperate to avoid losing the house I rented, my dad had helped me secure a bankruptcy attorney. So another anniversary low-point came during my appearance before a bankruptcy judge where I sat in a federal courtroom looking up at him from my wheelchair. For someone who loved to work and had always been proud of her independence, the humiliation was suffocating. I sat there in front of a room packed with others waiting their turn to do the same thing and rehashed what had happened to me. My petition for Chapter 7 bankruptcy was granted, which gave me more or less a clean slate for my financial collapse up to that point. However, it could do nothing for what was yet to come.

At times, I still thought I could use mind over matter to stop the hemorrhaging. I continued to try to work as many hours as I could in an effort to prove it was possible. I was proud to have almost worked 40 hours one week, but doing it was so exhausting that I was unable to do much of anything the next week. It seemed the more I tried to do to save what was left of my life, the worse my symptoms got.

I no longer felt safe living alone with my dogs and was realizing that if I continued to get worse, or even if stayed the same, I was in big trouble. Not having a name for my disease did nothing to slow down its progression, and I needed to find a way to stay with my dogs through whatever happened next. The fear I felt over not knowing what I had never subsided, but I knew it was time to stop obsessing over what it could be. Instead, I had to shift my focus. What I needed was to figure out how to be and what to do next.

As a therapist working with the homeless, I was aware of services available to them. Having been in Florida a relatively short time, I was a bit less familiar with services here than I would have liked, particularly for those with a physical disability. I called all of the resources listed in phone directories and in the Social Service directories I had used in my job. I did Internet searches and followed up on any leads I found there. The fact was, I was a single woman with no children and no diagnosis. I refused to believe that there was no help for me, so I continued to call, meet with and plead with agencies for assistance.

My landlord at the time also could not believe there was no help available, so I agreed to let her take me to several offices in another county where she believed they could help me. However, she saw for herself that there was no help. The phone calls and visits to agencies that are supposedly there to help were both futile and exasperating.

I am not just talking about financial aid. I am talking about getting wheelchair ramps put in or having my living space modified to make daily living easier. The bottom line was that if I had children or a diagnosis, I likely could have gotten help. I did manage to get myself placed on housing lists that were specific wheelchair housing and another waiting list for in-home assistance. I was still on those waiting lists seven years later when I had my name removed. I was told at many of the agencies that when I get a diagnosis, the organizations affiliated with the specific disease might be able to offer more.

Meanwhile, I was not able to work enough to pay rent, utilities and mounting medical bills. I briefly considered a move to my dad's home but his house has no spare room and the bedrooms are all upstairs, which would have been inaccessible for me. Another deal breaker for that option was that I would not have been able to keep my dogs. A couple different coworkers and I discussed a possible living arrangement where I could keep my dogs, but as each of those got closer to reality, they just did not work out.

I kept looking but met only dead ends. Each time I found a new agency or stumbled upon new information, I would have some hope that it was going to be okay. Each time someone wanted to help, I was again hopeful. Each time things fell through, I was crushed. If I needed money in the past, I would just work more. If I needed something done around the house, I would find out how and do it myself. I had always been able to figure things out and head off any major situation or loss. But this looked more and more like a train headed for a crash, and there was absolutely nothing I could do to stop it.

Then something unexpected happened, something that would soak this odyssey of mine in irony and take me somewhere I never would have expected to go.

I placed a phone call to chat with some of my former colleagues at the Homeless Emergency Project, the place I had loved to work and felt I was able to truly help so many homeless clients. I had just wanted to let everyone know how I was doing and update them on my situation. I was caught off guard when they suggested I could come live in one of their new, wheelchair accessible apartment units as a part of their Shelter Plus care program. I would not be able to keep my dogs, but they wanted me to know it was an option.

When the idea was first mentioned, I could only think that I still had not exhausted every avenue to find another place of my own where I could still have my dogs with me. But I am not sure why I thought that because I had already done that and was out of ideas. I think the truth is I just could not wrap my brain around the possibility of living in the same homeless housing project where just 12 months earlier I had placed my clients and saw them for therapy. I wanted to cover my head with my blanket and hide.

I had placed the call while lying on my bed and, as usual, Duke and Amore' were up there with me, blissfully unaware of the drama that was unfolding. They were my only solace amid the turmoil that was burning me like a wildfire. They each helped me in their own little ways. It was about this time that the deep bond I already had with them got deeper. They were two years old now and not only seemed to sense my loss of mobility; they actually stepped in to help me.

When I would fall and had trouble getting up, Duke was there, bracing himself to help me get to a place where I could get back up off the floor. When I was choking and gagging at night, they both licked my face, waking me so I could catch my breath. After I got the wheelchair and was unable to wheel it back up the driveway from the mailbox, they pulled me back up to the door. Amoré was the best at helping me find a comfortable position in bed when everything on my body was in constant spasm and hurting. He was not as squirmy as Duke was in bed, so my arm could rest comfortably at the perfect height of his body. I had tried different combinations of pillows, but nothing was as helpful as my Amoré. He is also the one that taught me to regulate my breathing and later on to meditate. When my arm was resting on his body at night, I would begin to breathe in sync with his relaxed breathing. These were the only times I could sleep.

So I could never give up on my commitment to them, nor could I fathom why I would want to get up each morning if it wasn't to take care of them. As I pulled them close to me and drank up the unmistakable love in their eyes, I renewed my quest to find another place to live, somewhere with wheelchair access, somewhere cheap and somewhere I could have my dogs. But I soon realized my quest had turned desperate when I began looking into the same seedy trailer parks where some of my former clients had lived. Just about everywhere I had tried, I was told my dogs were too big, and in the price range I could afford, none of the places had wheelchair ramps.

What was really going on was me stubbornly trying to avoid the reality that I wasn't getting any better. I was not going to wake up and find out I was dreaming. It was not until I let that sink in that I began to think more clearly. Even if I found a dump to live with the boys, what would happen if I got worse? What good would I be to my dogs then? Should I even be looking for a place to live when I no longer felt safe living alone? It was also becoming evident that if I had to cut my hours any more than I already had, I would have to file for Social Security Disability Insurance. And despite how much I wanted it not to be, the apartment at the homeless project was looking like my only option.

If I did move there --now more a matter of when than if--I needed to start brainstorming about where I could house my dogs, still be able to visit them and take them back when I could get my own place again. I found programs that would take them in but after checking deeper learned I would be surrendering ownership of them and they would be rehomed. I definitely was not going to do that.

Then, despite some uneasiness I had about the idea, I thought my landlord would provide the bridge I needed. She offered to keep them, figuring I would go to the shelter program, start getting disability income and then be able to get another place of my own. Like her, I was certain living at HEP would be temporary, although I also knew deep down that I could not really be sure of anything anymore.

The uneasiness I felt about her offer stemmed from her sometimes-erratic behavior. She would share with me some of her ideas for businesses, start to pursue them and then would drop them entirely. I just was not sure I could trust her with my dogs, either. She did not have a fenced yard, and I shuddered at the thought of them getting loose and being struck by a car.

The little voice in my head told me I needed a Plan B, and it was good that I listened.

My insurance policy would be my boss, Dan, who had always been so supportive. Not surprisingly, he said he would help. Less than 24 hours of asking him, my landlord backed out of the entire thing and asked me to leave the house before she returned from a trip two weeks later.

Her abrupt change of heart came the day after she had met someone who practiced alternative medicine. The next night she became insistent that I call him at the moment. It was late, I was in pain and exhausted and told her that I could not do one more thing that day. The truth was that I wanted to talk to him and I shared as much, but I couldn't do it that night. She took that as a slap in the face and sent me an email telling me as much, adding that I was an ungrateful, unmotivated person who no longer deserved to be helped because I was not helping myself. Ouch. Was I all of that? I did not really know what or who I was anymore. People closest to me assured me I was none of those things. I wasn't convinced and was feeling beaten down and tired of it all.

So, plan B it was. Dan would keep the boys, hopefully for a very temporary period and I would proceed to file for disability while living in the homeless program and working 12 hours/week. I would see the boys as often as we could coordinate it.

After I was sure that I had exhausted all possible alternatives, and essentially being evicted from my house, I finally surrendered as much as I could to the idea of going to live at the homeless project, which meant I would have to go there to fill out paperwork and set a move-in date.

A friend from work drove me there to take care of it. It was good she wasn't someone I knew well enough to open up to about my thoughts and feelings. The ride would be a quiet one. The only sounds were in my head and in my guts, my brain trying to outrun what was going on and my stomach twisting and churning like a kid walking home with a bad report card. It was a reality beyond my ability to process. I could not describe how I was feeling because it was different from anything I had ever felt before.

I know my dogs were on my mind and that as soon as I set a move-in date at HEP, I would have to do the same for them. I could not catch my breath. I needed to stop and regroup. When I was a little girl, I used to call "time-out" during games with my friends. When I would have bad dreams, I would shout "time-out" in my sleep because I just needed a break from the scary parts. In my head, I was still screaming and begging for a "time-out"

I cannot tell you how many times I drove a client over to the homeless program to complete the same paperwork I was about to fill out. I never gave a second thought to how they were feeling about signing up to live at a homeless program. If I did think about it, I would have just presumed they would be grateful to have a place to go. I was grateful for a place to go, but there was so much more to what I was feeling than gratitude, and I was not even sure I could express what that was.

I tried to express it in an email to my first real Florida friend, a woman named Karen who I worked with at the same Mental Health Center. During the first year of my illness, she and her husband, Bradford, had always been there to lend emotional support and do whatever they could to help me. She would do my laundry or even come over to open bottles and jars for me when I could not make my hands do it. Her husband mowed my lawn, and once laid bags of cement in the pouring rain along my fence line to keep my dogs from digging out of the yard.

Here are the emails Karen and I exchanged later on my sign-in day:

Dan says he is ok with dogs as long as it is temporary. God I hope it is a temporary separation. Anyway, he will take them Friday [July] 30th after work and I will spend first night at the HEP apartment Friday night also. Will be interesting weekend for me for so many reasons. His house isn't accessible for me, so not sure how visiting dogs will go....I tried to prolong going to set this date because the thought of going to make it more real was making me want to puke... The closer we got to HEP, the more I felt sure I was going to hurl. She [coworker] just kept asking me why I was so anxious--tried only once to explain and just shut up. Staff at HEP were a bit more validating and understood why and said they would be there for me for whatever I needed. Feel sick still. I am their client now, not coworker, colleague or friend. So bizarre I have no way to sort the feelings out or express them. All I can say is that I want to puke thinking about it, cry, and ask God what the f*%# else he wants from me, etc... Am sure it will be ok at some point but this is too weird for words. Think I am sort of in shock about it. We went after and got storage unit.

Met my roomie---older woman, no teeth, seemed nice though. Apartment is nice; one bedroom is small and will be interesting to see what it is like with power chair. I now have more to do---since I have date set...now I have to figure out what the hell to do with everything and figure out who can help pack and when. You are welcome as well but you would have to just be tissue holder and hugger. I cannot believe this. I really cannot believe it. What in the world is going on here? I have now lost everything?! Hung on for more than a year to the dogs, house, and pseudo full-time employment. Wow, really must be in another world or on another planet, right? Am I psychotic and don't know it and this really isn't happening?

    I will say that this life is quite entertaining from a distance, but not so much up close. I am going to work tomorrow. I may need time next week or week after and need to pretend I have reasons to get up right now and keep going. Sleeping sucks, waking sucks. Jeez, well, I am a bummer. Sorry. I am stunned. I am scared. I am angry. I am sad. In sum freaked out!!!!!...Housing will alleviate some of stressors I have now. This will calm down; I know this but I sure am not there yet. Just have to get through this part because there has to be a reprieve after all this.

    Response from Karen:

    Hi, you know the sick feeling you described...feeling like you needed to puke before, during, and after your visit to your apt... I actually get that. I think I am having sympathetic pains as I read the email. It had to be tough. I mean I am glad you have a home. And I do believe that the staff there will be there for you in any capacity. It is just the bizarreness of you having to be there and not as the co-worker or colleague. I am sick that you have lost so much, and yet quite impressed that you have not needed to be hospitalized through this for either emotional or physical. It is overwhelming from where I sit...really can't imagine your world and the only bright spot is you have a home and the dogs have a home. Shock is probably a good place to be...it will allow you to get stuff done.

    Stunned, scared, angry, sad and freaked out...yes, you are feeling all that. How could you not. Your friend feels all that too for you. I'll see you at work.~K

    My response back to Karen:
    I don't like sympathy pains Karen---I wish there was some

way everyone else could be immune to all of this...another negative to having others there for me? Anyway, I am sorry you get to participate in all of this. Am glad you are there and at the same time just wish, it had no impact on others. It is true, I have a home and boys have a home. Boys are with Dan and in good hands and I too am in good hands... Not done fighting, tired for sure, but with temporary framing to get boys back, I will fight for that for now. Get it where I can. Just counting on it slowing down soon so I can rest up for whatever comes after that. Again, I do wish that somehow you were immune to this and am sorry you are not. I really appreciate you Karen. You mustn't forget you are my hero anyway. I'll see ya later.

    In the final days at my house with my dogs, some of my friends from work were there to help me pack. I had a storage unit for some of my stuff, donated a lot, and the rest went out to the curb for the garbage. Keep in mind that I was hardly able to bathe routinely, so packing was not something that was happening very quickly. I donated a good portion of my furniture to HEP for its other units and many clothes went to its thrift store. I got rid of my referee uniforms and everything that represented physical activity because it seemed clear to me at the time that I would not need them again. Packing them up made me angry. These things only reminded me of what I was unable to do anymore.

    I was angry, sad, scared and feeling hopeless. I was moving into the same homeless program where many of my former and current clients still lived--right in the same apartment building. I did not mind so much about that, but I did mind moving there and losing my independence, my privacy and what seemed like my entire life, as I knew it. I had no idea what would happen next and I was less than eager to find out.

8

    I am not sure I knew how to feel or what to think when it was time to leave my home for the last time. A lot of stuff from the house was now in a heap by the curb, a pile some of my coworkers had to work their way around while they loaded my power chair into the truck. They were charged with taking me to live at the homeless project. My dogs had already moved, and right about then I sure could have used some doggie kisses to get through the rest of this day.

    During the 30 minutes or so it took to get there my brain was trying to make sense of the whirlwind of changes that had taken place in the past week alone. I tried to joke in the truck, but my humor had turned dark and dry. I seemed to be having trouble catching my breath and felt like I was repeatedly being kicked in the stomach.

    Apparently, it was big news that I was arriving because when we pulled into the parking lot about 6 p.m. it seemed like everyone who lived there was outside to greet me. I love an audience now, but then, not so much. We were entering my very own twilight zone. After emptying the truck and getting me back into the power wheelchair, my coworker friends said good-bye, and drove away. And there I sat, face-to-face with my new reality.

    Because I couldn't process all of what had happened in last 48 hours, I tried to just be present in the moment. I was still having trouble catching my breath. Breaking down and crying seemed appropriate and what I felt like doing, but it wasn't an option because I needed to be settled enough and unpacked enough to go to bed. I wondered when I would finally get to have that meltdown I had been staving off so long. It seemed there just was not a right time to lose it.

I made small talk with some of the residents and my new roommate, who was a sweet older woman named Caroline. Caroline helped me set up my elevated potty-chair and shower bench. We then had to coordinate space because there were two twin beds in the bedroom and my power chair had to be parked beside mine, so that I could get in and out of the bed. The chair also needed to be charged through the night, so wherever I parked it had to be near a wall plug. The space between the beds was only wide enough for my power chair, which meant she could not walk past it.

We tried a couple of different arrangements and none of them was great, so we decided to sleep on it and figure it out the next day. That first night, I was feeling insecure about not knowing my surroundings and was afraid I would not be able to get back into my chair to go to the bathroom in the middle of the night. Caroline pretty much let me do whatever I needed to do to feel comfortable.

Once I was at least somewhat settled, I ventured outside for a smoke. Just about everyone there smoked and those who didn't were out there with the smokers anyway. I had tried to quit several times since I had been working with the homeless, but because so many of them are smokers, it made it all the harder to stop.

The popular smoking area was behind the apartment building but as smoking areas go this one was primo. It was in a shaded area next to a kidney shaped estuary about the size of a couple football fields. The water's edge closest to the apartment was lined with a wave of lush green reeds that rose a few feet into the air and swayed in even the hint of a summer breeze. It was really just a big pond that fed into a creek that meandered its way west a few miles west where it emptied into the Intracoastal Waterway.

But nestled where it was and circled by a canopy of palm trees and sprawling oaks whose branches cast a tarp of welcome shade, it was an oasis, its water a jewel that got its glitter from the sun. I had been there many times before with clients, mixing equal doses of therapy and cigarettes. But on this day, I found out that even a smoke break was something I could no longer take for granted.

I took the wheelchair ramp that zigzagged down from my second floor apartment to a sidewalk next to a rolling grass area that led the smoking area about 50 feet away. So there I sat, stuck on the sidewalk at the bottom the ramp with no way of getting my wheelchair over to where everybody was waiting. The way my body and emotions reacted to this roadblock was pretty intense and while I held it together externally, I secretly wondered if this would be the final straw that breaks me entirely.

I tearfully sat over by the ramp and lit a cigarette. Some of the people who lived there started gathering pieces of scrap plywood to improvise a ramp from the sidewalk over the grass so that I could join them. It took a while but they managed to get me over there. It would be the first of many times that the people there, my neighbors and former clients, would find a solution to give me access to something that seemed out of reach.

It felt about 15 degrees cooler under the trees by the water, an arctic blast for me since I found the extreme Florida heat almost intolerable. That little estuary was beautiful to me that first night and my spirits were buoyed when I saw that it was home to a wonderful assortment of waterfowl and fish.

I decided to distract myself by engaging others in conversations that didn't leave me vulnerable and talking about myself on my first night there. Everyone knew I was the homeless outreach therapist turned homeless woman in a wheelchair. I am not sure what else everyone knew for sure, but everyone seemed to be gathered around me. For a while, I pretended that I was at work and was able to maintain composure and interact effectively and appropriately with everyone.

It was too hard to think about not having even a shred of what was once my life, but I refused to break down while my thoughts drifted from what the others were sharing. I wondered if coffee and cigarettes would be enough to get me out of bed in the morning. My motivation to get up and keep moving forward was always my dogs, and I had serious doubts I would be able to motivate myself. While I had them only three years, my dogs had become my reason for living when I could not come up with other good enough reasons. They got me to a new therapist when I moved to Florida and they were the ones who made me consider my own safety over the past year. I did it all for them to ensure they were taken care of the best way I could take care of them. Now I did not have them and was becoming increasingly worried about my emotional well-being.

My thoughts stopped drifting suddenly when I noticed that several of the residents were feeding the ducks. Perhaps, I thought, I would also feed the ducks since they come around mostly in the mornings and in evenings, about the same times I would normally be feeding Duke and Amore.

Within a week, I had a dog visit schedule set up for every other Saturday, had taken charge of the duck feeding, and had figured out that the only time I could be alone was early in the mornings before the sun came up. I discovered the first morning there that I had a new love—the great blue heron. It took me a bit longer to learn more about the great blue, and to figure out that there were two of them living together in a tree on the other side of the estuary.

One of them, the female I believe, turned out to be a magnificent messenger, teaching me to balance being a solitary and social being. She also was urging me to reflect on my internal feelings and beliefs so that I could re-evaluate them. She could hunt her prey without making so much as a ripple in the shallows. That fascinated me. I was also amazed that I had never noticed this bird in what used to be my very busy life. I was never still in my life and generally kept as busy as I could to avoid stillness. Now, stuck in a wheelchair, I had been forced to be still, and was seeing my world from a completely different place.

I had been at HEP for 12 days, and I still was unable to reconcile how my life had gone from one thing to another so quickly. I snatched some time alone that day and wrote an entry in my journal:

Trying to find moment of pure peace right now and pen and

paper historically have been my best way to achieve that. Writing is harder now, but I am drawn to the page lately. James Taylor is singing in my headphones while I try to hide in the shade behind the building under the A/C units. Otherwise someone always wants to talk to me, regardless of what I may be doing at the time. I am at HEP's Shelter Plus care program and my dogs are with Dan. A hurricane is moving in end of the week and I only want to be with Duke and Amore. I miss them with all my heart right now. I have never missed anyone or anything more in my life. My heart is so tied to them and I am at a loss without them. Now my responsibilities are only me and work.

    I am slowly adjusting to this fact. I have seen the boys weekly though. I have so many mixed feelings—a hodge-podge of intensity-laden ones. I am doing well not staying in the mess of feelings though. Thankful for the new day to start it over. In spite of so many many many losses incurred in past year and half, I find myself grateful for so much. I am so open to the lessons and opportunities for growth because part of me knows one of two things is inevitable. 1) I will only get worse and may lose my ability to communicate effectively, or 2) I will get really bad and die soon. As scary as those both seem, I have to have things in order so that I get undone things done and dead issues buried. The communication with my ex and his parents was very important to me. Although brief, it was so important to get where I can work on that and forgive myself. They do, they say God does and I have to get there soon.

    I am more focused on telling the people who have been pivotal in my life that I appreciate them. I need them to know that, even though I was not really able to express it back then. I have many of them to thank as so many have come and gone at key times in my life. Dan gets irritated when I tell him thank you all the time, but I don't care really. God has something in mind for me. I wonder sometimes what the hell else he wants from me in this life. I am angry at God—mostly because I don't get it. I am more still than ever, but this move is too new to focus on what spirit tells me. Am sure I miss signs all over so far. Maybe I'll get it soon. All I ask is to have quality of life and hope the dogs are in the cards for me to have along the way. God knows how I am and maybe he separated us to teach me something? To show me how to better find my purpose from within? He knows my drive is not so much for me, but for the boys. They have taught me so much and all of those lessons have been reinforced by becoming disabled. All that I was working on has come to me easier since getting worse.

    I remain present more often than not, which I consider a miracle. I miss things/abilities I had. I miss basketball and running with the boys. Right now with this living situation, I miss privacy. I cannot isolate because I smoke cigarettes and there is no chance to not interact with others if you smoke. 8-11-2004 THSC

    I was still racking up more symptoms with the passing days, so my morning private time in the gentleness of sunrise by the water seemed to help keep me sane. Feeding the ducks made me feel somehow useful and needed. I had a purpose. I was working 12 hours a week in the Day Treatment Program at Directions and attempting to navigate the Social Service system during the day. Somehow, I could shift my thoughts to look forward to this time with the great blue, as long as I had a visit coming up with my dogs. I was amply distracted from my pain and circumstances by becoming entranced in the other residents' stories about how they ended up there. I have always loved a great story.

9

    They say that when you are dying your life passes before your eyes. I may not have been about to take my last breath but the possibility I might not live much longer haunted me and those flashbacks of my life often came to me in the stillness of the sunrises and sunsets by the water.

    The images flipped through my head as if my brain was thumbing through the pages of a book. There were distant replays of moments from my childhood like climbing trees behind our house or trying to keep up with my older brother and his friends playing kickball in our front yard in the shade of a giant weeping willow. I'm the little cheerleader in the navy blue and white uniform getting in trouble for watching the basketball game instead of cheerleading. There I am playing Dukes of Hazard with my friend Kelly in a neighbor's parked car. And there I am wading in a country creek with friends looking for crawdads. There are flashes of me in high school, playing point guard on the basketball team and running relays in track. There I am hiking to the top of a ridge to sit on a boulder and imagine living a different life. I see faces of people I used to know and others whose names I can't remember.

    But the flashbacks that were clearest were from my college days, the way I came to find a career path, my battle with eating disorders and depression, and more than all that came the images of my alcoholic mother who died at 46, the one person I wanted so desperately to please and was so unable to save.

    The glimpses of my life rolled through my mind with a shroud of darkness as a backdrop, the foreboding that was the cornerstone of my depression. But I was able to fight it back and let in flickers of light that came from the certainty I clung to that life had something more in store for me. I was trying to find the bigger picture, even though what was in front of me was looking worse than it ever had. My illness had been teaching me lessons about control, asking for help and confronting my vulnerabilities. I was sure I had more to learn about all that, but what did I have to learn by losing my dogs and living with the very population I was so passionate to serve? How in the world did I ever end up living in a homeless project?

Now, sitting outside in my wheelchair under the hum of an air conditioning and watching a blue heron, I had time to trace the journey that brought me there, the highs and lows spread out like pieces of a puzzle:

I was a journalism major when I went to college because I wanted to write about things that matter. My dream was to be able to embed myself into situations as an investigative reporter and then write about what I experienced. I even got a job in high school at a pet store so that I could monitor how the animals were treated. It was important to me to know that the animals were getting out of the cages and their cages were clean. It turned out my job was the cage cleaner and the one who got them out of their cages, so there really was no story there.

Along with journalism, I enjoyed my psychology courses. But at the time I went to college, I didn't really want to be that close to uncovering the very issues I struggled with internally. My mom stuff was not ready to be confronted yet. I figured I could just write human-interest stories and that would satiate my interest in the field of psychology. I could never have imagined that someday I would be writing a story both as a homeless advocate and therapist and as someone who became homeless.

By my sophomore year, I was really struggling. I had an eating disorder since high school and it was starting to catch up to me. I was working as a student assistant with the Student Health Education Program at the time and did a story for the university newspaper about eating disorder awareness. By this time, I was miserable and I could not stop binging and purging on my own. I had been trying to stop but could not.

I decided to get some help and actually knew how to do that

since I had gathered all of that information for my story. What I didn't know was that help would involve me being admitted to an inpatient facility for nearly two months. I didn't think I was that bad. During the treatment, I was also diagnosed with depression, and though I knew I was depressed all throughout my childhood, I denied it. I found out that it was actually the eating disorder that was helping me cope with the depression, but I did not understand that at the time.

To go into treatment, I had to withdraw from my courses for medical reasons. I had spent years hiding my behavior and now I was having to tell people about it. I wished I could just go hide in treatment and then make up something about where I had been.

But, as it turned out, it was the treatment program that redirected my career path. Once I got through it, I decided I might want to pursue psychology. I had seen good therapists and I had seen bad therapists during my treatment. I wanted to be one of the good ones who genuinely cared about the patient. I had been exposed to group therapy and thought I did well diverting attention from myself and asking the other patients questions. I waited for a couple of semesters to decide change my major to psychology.

In my junior year, I had a health crisis that ended with a lymph node biopsy, but no one could quite figure out why I was so fatigued and weak. I had to take a few incompletes. Between that and the eating disorder treatment, I was on the five-year plan to graduate with my bachelor's degree. I was working part time, going to school full time, and was just tired of being in school by the time it was nearly over. I was going to get married and had a promotion at work once I graduated, so I already had a lot going on in 1994. So much so, that instead of getting married in May, we decided to wait until August. I very much wanted my mom to see me get married and it seemed she might be running out of time.

Graduate school would wait two years because between work and school, I was also running back and forth to tend to my mother who loved to call me in a drunken crisis. I always went to her to try to help when she called. She was in bad shape from the alcohol and had almost died many times since I was a freshman in high school. She nearly died the week she was scheduled to come for a family session when I was in treatment. I never knew which time I went to see her would be the last time.

I was tired of school, but mostly postponed graduate school because I didn't want to commit to a program knowing that it was unlikely my mother would live much longer. She died on December 30 in 1995 in the ICU. I struggled for months after her death. My heartache over losing her was compounded because I had always made my decisions based on what she wanted for me. That weighed heavily on my mind when I decided to apply to graduate school that spring to study clinical psychology at Marshall University. Would she approve? Would this decision finally make her like me? I was sure that pursuing clinical psychology was what I wanted to do. I was also sure she did not like therapists since she told me they would brainwash me when I went to treatment myself.

I concluded it was what I should have done when I first went to college. Much to my surprise, I was accepted into the graduate program that fall, partly because some of those who were selected declined. The program only accepted 12 applicants each year, so even though it was somewhat by default, I was still proud to get in.

Fast forward to graduating from the clinical psychology program, the honor of working at the hospital where I had been in treatment, a divorce, the program closing at the hospital. Long story later, and I was having some problems finding a job. I worked a few different part-time jobs, became a basketball referee and worked on an eating disorder book that I never finished.

It was time to find full time work again, so I was applying for just about anything. I applied for a position as a substance abuse/mental health therapist at the Men's Emergency Shelter program about an hour away. I got an interview. I almost didn't go because I was sure I wouldn't want to work there. I was hired and was excited because my boss was turning this shelter into a program that was providing many different services--not just shelter and basic case management. It would later be renamed the Roark-Sullivan Lifeway Center (RSLC) and I would get to be a part of helping develop new programs and grants under a wonderful mentor. I got to learn about grant writing, grant management, program development and most of all just how human homeless men really are.

I was moved by the homeless men there at the shelter, loved hearing how they ended up there, and was struck by how one decision or two created the consequences that led them to homelessness. It seemed it could happen to anyone—even me. I had former professors, doctors, professionals of all kinds, all education levels, as clients there.

A relationship I had been in was coming to an end, which led me to make my decision to move myself and my dogs to Florida. My father moved to Florida when I went to college, my brother and his family followed dad there after mom died, and I was the last to arrive in March of 2002. I was 31, had been married and divorced and was running away from another relationship. I had a niece and a half brother and sister whose lives I really wanted to be a part of, so I came down and after finding a job, went back and got my dogs.

I had applied for several different types of jobs before landing a position as a homeless outreach therapist. I followed some signs on my way to scope out dog parks, found a house to rent, and took a weekend drive to pick up my dogs.

Soon after that, I got a call to interview for an adjunct teaching position I had applied for at St. Petersburg College. I got the job, joined a basketball officials association, and had recreated the same life I had in West Virginia. Only this time I was single, living alone with my two dogs, and my family was only a few miles away.

I even had a couple of homeless clients from the shelter in West Virginia show up in Florida. The joke with the staff and clients at one of the local homeless providers was that they were my groupies.

I was devoted to helping the homeless, and in Florida I worked with both men and women clients. I loved working in the field and collaborating with the different service providers to advocate for what my clients needed. Through my work with the homeless, I came to truly believe that most people, myself included, were a paycheck or two away from being homeless too. I also came to understand that they were the human population without a voice. They were invisible to most people because to see them would mean they would have to also recognize themselves in each one. They were often dismissed and considered throwaways. If anyone would meet any of the hundreds of people I worked with who happened to be homeless, they could surely see that they were once professionals who had lives, had the house in the suburbs with the 2.5 kids and a dog.

They were not any different than the rest of us. Some got hurt working on a job that didn't pay workman's compensation. Some went through divorces or their spouses died. Some took care of a dying relative and other family members pushed them out of the will. Others had undiagnosed mental illnesses such as depression or bipolar disorder and ended up addicted to a substance that they started out using to self-medicate. Others had physical illnesses they didn't have medical insurance to treat, lost their job, and the physical illness got worse.

The people I would see on the street and those that are referred to as the "street homeless" were once productive members of society. They tried to get on their feet shortly after becoming homeless, but were unable to, and the services they needed weren't accessible. After a while, they turned to alcohol or they turned to complete isolation, so living outdoors where no one bothered them was preferable to a shelter environment. We see them and say things like, "They choose to remain homeless" or "They put themselves there." That couldn't be further from the truth. There is always so much more to each story than what we see on the surface. It was those stories that kept me getting up and working 14 -16 hour days. It was their invisibility to others that drove me to educate and advocate on their behalf. It was the challenge of uncovering so many layers of issues that made my job so compelling.

Of course, I also knew that my drive was wearing me out. I was driven by more than those people right in front of me who needed me. It really wasn't about whoever was in crisis that day or my current clients. I was essentially trying to save my mother over and over again with each one. I couldn't save my mom from herself, but I seemed determined to continue to try even long after her death. This was a powerful realization I had before my illness started, and one that allowed me to slow down a bit at work, and to remove some of the pressure I was putting on myself. I felt that I failed my mom because I couldn't save her from herself. I had no idea I felt this way or that this was my motivation. I realized this about four months before my symptoms began.

Also during the months before my symptoms started, I had been making strides toward improvements in mood and in continuity between my behaviors and my priorities.

I first encountered the Homeless Emergency Project while working with Directions for Mental Health. We worked with a police homeless outreach team, which identified homeless from the streets and helped coordinate services with the two therapists to get them off the streets.

As with most not-for-profit work, the hours were long and the work challenging. I saw clients at the soup kitchen, the beach, local parks and just about anywhere they were. I loved the work and grew quite fond of the staff of all of the service providers. The staff at HEP was mostly women, nurturing women. It always felt good to interact with them while I was seeing clients there, and they seemed to give my clients and me the benefit of the doubt. I trusted they would work well with my clients and they trusted I was doing all that I could to ensure my clients were working toward getting better and following the rules.

When my symptoms began, I struggled getting around to different places. I was backing my car into things because my right leg didn't always have the strength to push down the brake. I had to stop transporting clients. It was a challenge to drive, but also a challenge to get to where the clients were and to spend the time doing therapy with them. I had seen many of them for at least a couple of months and they too seemed to be concerned about my deteriorating health.

From my outreach work, as I was continuing to accrue more symptoms, I changed positions to work at a long-term substance abuse, mental health and homeless program at another partner program. The homeless outreach grant was ending and not being applied for again, so it made sense to try to get the clients I had into this program because what was most missing was the long term, residential treatment setting that included the understanding of homelessness. It was my dream job. In my very brief tenure there, I continued to work with the staff at HEP where some of my former clients were on waiting lists for the long-term program.

When I was again transferred to different position because my symptoms had continued to limit the number of hours I was able to work, I still kept in touch with the HEP staff because some of my Day Treatment clients were living there and had also been my clients out in the field.

Progressively sidelined by my illness, I had lasted nearly a year from that last job change before having to let go of my dogs and become a homeless statistic. Through it all, my compassion for the homeless never wavered. I always took the time to listen to their stories. They came back to see me. They made progress. They would regress. They would come back. They knew I genuinely cared about what happened to them. And I did. I still do. It is just that their story had become my story. I was them. They were me.

That is how I got here, the woman in the wheelchair watching her life flash through her mind.

I had always told my clients that it could be me or anyone else in their shoes. Most people don't like to admit it—I said it myself, but never thought it would actually happen to me.

It wasn't surprising that despite my attempts to resist it, my inner darkness cast its shadow over me with growing regularity. It was in those dark places that I would dwell on whether I was going to be able to live much longer, especially without my dogs. I missed Duke's watchful eyes looking out for me, and my armrest at night that was Amoré. I was scared of choking to death at night without them there to wake me. I was living for them, consumed with finding a way we could somehow, some way be reunited.

So there I was, stripped of all that was once my life, without my boys there to give me motivation to go on, haunted by frightening doubts that I would care enough to keep getting up in the morning.

But I did get up. I fed the ducks, watched the great blue herons and the water. I struggled with pain, with sleep, with darkness. Some nights were particularly dark and each time I went to see my neurologist, it only got darker. My chart still said rule-out the terminal disease amyotrophic lateral sclerosis (ALS) – known as Lou Gehrig's disease -- as my working diagnosis. That scared me sick and made me want to look at my life and all that was left undone and unsaid. I had to look at what I had created through the years and sabotaged, then what I newly created and lost altogether. I looked at all that I had planned to do and hadn't gotten around to doing yet. I had lost things and people in my life before, but never had I literally lost everything. I was not sure if I was about to lose my life too.

The pain tormented me, my leg and arm muscles felt like they were so tight that they could break my bones, depriving me of sleep while I screamed inside for it to please stop. I'm not sure how, but I kept getting up in the morning, and my worsening symptoms and the pain got up with me. There would be more medication but none of it brought much relief. It got so I could no longer handle anyone having any expectations of me. It seemed everything I did or tried to do was a failure, so I couldn't seem to commit too much. If I committed, it would turn out I could not do it anyway because of pain or fatigue or something else.

I could commit to the expectations of the ducks. They expected me to feed them and I did. I could also handle my visits with my dogs. They expected me to love on them and savor each and every second in their energy and presence, and I did.

10

The spot where I parked myself, next to the water with my bag of bird seed for the ducks and my pack of Marlboros, had become my sanctuary. I found solace in that patch of green and blue, so soothing in morning mists and creeping dusks. I had tried to keep the borders of my world small, my apartment, my ramp, my cigarettes, my ducks, my herons, my thoughts. Of course, where I lived was no isolation booth, and my pristine, little oasis seemed somehow misplaced.

Just beyond the north edge of the water and in full view and earshot of where we smoked, stood a crack house, the hub of a neighborhood known for drugs and prostitution. It was a two-story, dilapidated clapboard house, pockmarked by weather-faded, peeling gray paint and broken windows. As the evenings wore on, it got busier and louder, much worse on weekends.

It was a somewhat fitting contrast, and it cast some irony on the location of the new HEP apartment I now called home. On one side, an estuary teeming with birds, fish and new life, on the other, blight. On one side, homeless people getting help and having hope. On the other side, hopelessness.

The piercing shrill of sirens was our constant companion with ambulances speeding along the main road toward a hospital three miles to the north. There was a fire station a half mile away, and police cars were commonplace in the disadvantaged neighborhood where crime and violence had long ago taken a foothold. About the only night sound I liked was the melancholy wail of a train whistle from the tracks just off to the south, stirring in me a longing to be on it going somewhere else, anywhere else.

It was amid those sights and sounds that HEP first plunked down roots in 1986 to help a growing homeless population in Pinellas County. From humble beginnings in a church called Everybody's Tabernacle, today its campus spans eight city blocks that contain a 10,000-square-foot main office building and resident service center, an eight-unit family shelter, a 32-unit apartment complex for veterans, a 16-unit apartment complex for the disabled, and the eight unit apartment for single adults where I was living.

My apartment building was built just a few months before I arrived and plans were already set to build a new thrift shop across the street to replace the old one that now stood framed by clusters of weeds and brush at the rear of a crumbling asphalt parking lot.

The apartments in my building were each one bedroom with twin beds. The wheelchair unit where I lived was a bit larger with a little more floor space in the kitchen and bathroom. A grand opening was scheduled a couple of months after I moved in and the handicap unit was the one they wanted to spotlight for the media.

I liked the idea and wanted to help my new roommate, Sue, clean the apartment and make it presentable for its public debut.

I just hadn't planned on hurting myself, having my former colleagues tour my place, and then be the focus of a newspaper article. I was excited for HEP to be expanding and wanted to do my part to make the unveiling a success. I did not think much beyond that, and apparently even less about my safety during the cleanup.

I had taken a broom and was swatting at cobwebs high in the corners of the living room. I could sort of stand if I was leaning against something sturdy while putting most of my weight on my left leg. The sole of my right foot had become twisted from its spastic muscles so I could only put weight on the backside of the heel. My left leg wasn't predictable or stable. It could go into spasm at any time, and would shake like crazy if the muscles were flexed or my leg was unexpectedly touched.

I spotted a cobweb in the far corner on the other side of the couch. I couldn't quite reach it with the broom while sitting in the wheelchair, so I decided to do my leaning routine to get at it. Stretching just out of reach of the cob web, I went down, landing sideways and horribly on part of the couch and part of the floor. I screamed in pain. My left foot was stuck in the footplate of the wheelchair and my lower body was twisted against the couch. My left leg was bent in the opposite direction, wrenching my left knee and ankle. After the tears subsided and Sue helped me back into my chair, I tried to assess the damage I had done. I was already on a potent pain patch and myriad other medications, which made it hard to gauge how much pain I was actually in. I opted to try to ignore it and deal with it after the big event.

In all the cleaning, rearranging and preparation for the opening, it did not occur to me that most of the people who would be touring my apartment were going to be colleagues. I did not fully grasp that until the morning of the event. They were some of the same people I had advocated to on behalf of my clients and met with regularly. Some were people I had not seen since before my illness began.

When I did realize who they were, I wanted to hide. How in the world was I supposed to react when these folks saw me sitting in a wheelchair, showing them my new apartment in a homeless project? What would I say? I wondered what protocol was for such a situation and then realized there was no protocol. I would just have to suck it up and be however I needed to be, sharing only what I needed to share.

Our place looked great. My newly hurt knee and ankle made transferring from the chair really challenging and both were hurting in spite of the pain medications already in my system. I would worry about that later. At that moment, I was becoming increasingly anxious about all of the people I knew parading through my apartment all day.

The next thing I knew, I was being interviewed by a newspaper reporter. I didn't know I was going to be one of the ones who would be interviewed and none of us knew which interviews would make the final cut for her article. So I was somewhat taken aback when I read the article and saw that I was quoted prominently. It hadn't occurred to me that this would be out there for God and everybody to see. What was I thinking? I worried about what my dad, step mom and brother would think about the story. Was I an embarrassment for them? Probably.

Embarrassment was surely among the emotions I had felt when I encountered so many colleagues that day, although mostly it just felt awkward. I shared what I had to share with them and they seemed to have an appreciation for my situation, especially given that my former clients were my neighbors. Many of them were surprised to see me and even more surprised to see me in a wheelchair. I still wasn't a fan of telling my story, but was able to do it that day in a fairly detached manner, almost as if it was telling someone else's story.

When it was over, I was exhausted, and not looking forward to figuring out how badly I had hurt myself in the cobweb fall.

The grand opening that turned out to be considerably less than grand for me was the first of two HEP experiences that summer that truly challenged my stubborn denial of my situation. The second came about a week later when the census takers came.

There is one day set aside each year for a nationwide homeless count. Each community puts together teams of people to count the homeless. They fan out to soup kitchens, shelters, parks, wooded areas, beaches and anywhere else the homeless could be found. In each of the previous three years, I was a homeless census team member. There was a form we had people fill out and sign, and they usually got a free t-shirt and some other goodies for their time.

I wasn't a part of the census team this time. I wasn't even aware it was That Day until I went outside the apartment for something and spotted a former colleague and my caseworker named Trish with t-shirts and a clipboard. I asked what was going on and she told me what I already knew. It was the homeless count and she asked if I would come down and fill out the form for her.

I stopped moving forward in my chair for just a moment because I was flashing back to the previous years of counting the homeless myself. Time stood still and I am not sure for how long, but I replied to Trish that I would be down in a minute.

That sensation of being kicked in the gut and losing my breath was getting to be a regular occurrence. I wondered if I would eventually get used to it. Each time it happened, I was so taken off guard that it would take me a few minutes or more to catch my breath and slow my heart rate back down. I had admitted to myself that I had become a homeless statistic the day I filled out the paperwork to move in there, but being asked by a census taker to come down and document it was so much harder to take. It now would be signed, sealed and undeniable that I was just like everyone else there, not an exception, not someone who just happened to be there but really shouldn't be. The real-ness of it all was about to hit me once again, tying another knot in my stomach and raising another lump in my throat.

I motored over to Trish quietly. I waited for the clipboard, filled out the form, signed my name and got my free t-shirt with some local business's logo on it. Holding the t-shirt as she handed it to me, I said, "Well, I guess that really makes it official, huh?" Trish wasn't sure what I meant, so I explained that I was officially a homeless outreach therapist turned homeless statistic today.. Her eyes changed as she looked at me. It hadn't occurred to her that it would be a big deal to sign a sheet of paper, but once I said that, her eyes filled with compassion and she gave me a big hug.

While I had slowed my heart rate some before going over to where Trish was in the parking lot, I had just increased it again and filled my eyes with tears by making such a statement aloud. Her hug seemed to make the tears want to spill over and down my face, so I said a quick thank you and motored away from everyone to avoid making a scene. I have never been a fan of crying in front of people, and this certainly was not the time or place for me to bawl my eyes out. I almost felt a bit silly because really I was already a homeless client, so that was nothing new. Signing a piece of paper didn't really change anything. Yet at the same time, it felt like everything changed.

11

    Somehow I was able to hold myself together emotionally for the grand opening and the census. I was good at that. No matter how something ripped at me on the inside, I could check myself and not show it outwardly. But there was one notable exception that homeless summer and it came in the form of a very large woman on a scooter.

    It happened soon after my worsening condition meant I had to give up the measly 12 hours a week I worked for Directions as a day treatment therapist. I was feeling so disconnected, useless and frustrated that I was an emotional perfect storm when they called a general meeting of all HEP clients a couple days later.

    The meeting was called to address the fact that many clients were not contributing the mandated 10 hours a week of volunteer work. It was really about the able-bodied, unemployed clients who were able to volunteer to do something and weren't, and not aimed at me specifically. But you couldn't have convinced me of that and my defenses were on full alert.

    I had stopped working because even 12 hours had become too much – even though all I had to do was sit and do therapy -- and now they were wanting me to do something for 10 hours. What could I do anymore? I felt the expectations were too high and I felt that the entire meeting was about me not volunteering my time.

    Did no one appreciate all of the crisis intervention and free therapy I was doing at the apartments? I wasn't doing it for recognition, rather because I could and it was often needed around there. I was the victim and martyr that day and I doubt there was anything anyone could have said or done that would have changed that mindset.

My dials were set on full boil when after the meeting I encountered an extremely obese client who had just taken delivery of a spanking new, red power scooter. The sight of her and the way she was carrying on, immediately reminded me how I had to fight my insurance company for several months to get a power wheelchair, even though I desperately needed it at the time.

She was perfectly capable of walking, but laughed about not having to anymore since she could get a scooter paid for through Medicaid. She had told everyone about it the week before when her doctor wrote the prescription for it. Here she was riding around on it as if it was a toy. My power chair had become my legs in the time I had spent in it so far, and to see someone playing on one made my blood boil. The sight of her with her new toy nearly pushed me over the edge, which that day was not far for me to go. I was so angry that I felt as though my head might pop off my neck.

She epitomized why the homeless and people using motorized mobility equipment are misunderstood. She had her issues, don't get me wrong, but she was not interested in working on them while she was living off HEP and the system. She didn't even want to have to put forth the effort to walk for herself. I was in victim mode, so I was viewing everything in terms of fair or unfair and most of what I was seeing in my personal situation was unfair. Here was someone who wasn't trying, was perfectly capable of walking, had no desire to get better or change her life and things were going smoothly for her. I was doing everything I could think of to survive from one day to the next and nothing was going right for me. It was a flashpoint, and I couldn't stop my rage from boiling over:

I couldn't censor my words. It was as if they were flowing out, and my mouth no longer knew how to close. At first, I was only venting to those around me who knew me the best—my roommate, the veteran, the fisherman. I thought I got it all out and calmed down a bit. Next thing I know, histrionic woman motors out of her apartment toward the ramp in her new scooter totally cutting me off from going the same direction. She was laughing about not having to do anything ever again, as if she were the queen on her new throne.

"That thing is not a f$%&-ing toy and I don't appreciate you acting like it is." I yelled angrily. She laughed at me. Yep, she laughed. She was large and I was puny and had more sense than to get into any kind of a battle with her, so I said nothing more. She could take me and wouldn't hesitate. I had never been in a fight in my life and this was not the best time to start. My first inclination was to motor after her in my chair, and that was what I did. In just a few feet, I played out the potential scenarios in my mind. I stopped when I realized that her scooter went faster than my power chair. Besides that, if she wanted to get out of her chair, she could outrun me on her own. I simply waited for my head to explode as I tried to calm down. She was one of the able-bodied people not volunteering in the community.

It was about an hour after my tantrum that I realized how ridiculous it had all been. My anger wasn't about her, or her scooter. It wasn't about how fast and easily she was able to get her scooter, either. It was just me taking out on her the layers of anger that had been caking up inside me since this damn disease started snatching away my life. I had plenty of anger to go around, some for the doctors and even some for God.

12

While it was true that my predicament had often left me wallowing in my darkest emotions that summer, flickers of the other me, the me I used to be, still bubbled up from time to time to remind me all was not lost. That was the me who loved to laugh, loved to have fun, loved an adventure, and most of the time loved life. She was the one who would go to any length to help somebody in need, and if it were an animal in trouble, all the better.

Take, for instance, the strange tale of a failed, but hilarious attempt to rescue an injured heron.

One evening, while the smokers' club was lingering by the water's edge, we collectively noted the odd behavior of one of the estuary's male Muscovy ducks, the one we had named Johnny. The general consensus was that Johnny wasn't too bright, particularly since he was constantly trying to mate with any duck he encountered regardless of whether it was a Muscovy. In fact, he left us wondering whether his mating appetite even included non ducks, which brings me to the heron.

We watched with great curiosity as the unsuspecting night heron, which had been wading innocently in a few inches of water, found itself caught in the throes of one of Johnny's mating frenzies. We weren't sure if Johnny was trying to mate with the heron or attacking it since both behaviors appeared to be similar where Johnny was concerned.

The flailing heron managed to get away but we noticed it may have broken a wing in the exchange because it was unable to fold it smoothly against its body like the other wing. I pulled the wheelchair over as far as I could along the bank in an attempt to follow it into the narrowing of the estuary, but never got close enough to see if it ever did get the wing to tuck in properly. Some of the others walked back there later but were unable to even spot it. But we collectively determined it was hurt and needed to be rescued.

The stage was set for an improbable, if not ill-advised adventure on the estuary with me of all people playing a starring role.

I got out a bird book that Sue, my roommate and co-conspirator, had scored some time earlier from the thrift store and determined that the injured bird was probably a black crested night heron. We showed the picture to others who had witnessed the tussle and they all agreed we had made a correct identification.

The idea of rescuing that bird fired me up at a time when I needed firing up. This was something I could do. I had spent a year and a half feeling useless and vowed that this would not be one of those times. I had spent my life trying to rescue humans and animals, and this time I wasn't going to let my wheelchair deter me.

We set the rescue operation in motion by calling the Suncoast Seabird Sanctuary which sent a woman out to talk to us about what happened. She told us that if we located the injured bird we could call her and she would come back to pick it up and take it to the sanctuary for treatment.

The next morning, Sue went to the thrift store and came back all excited with a box tucked under her arm. It was an inflatable raft that someone had donated and Sherry got it for us. It actually had sides on it and looked like a little rectangular, brown boat. I remember thinking my brother had one almost exactly like it when we were kids camping and boating back home on Sutton Lake. We reasoned it was exactly what we needed to get out in the water and hunt for the heron, and I insisted I would be part of the rescue mission, and I meant the in-the-raft part.

We didn't have an air pump, which meant that we had to inflate the raft by lung power. Since everyone was in on it, we all took turns until we got that raft full of air. That took most of the morning, but by mid-afternoon we were ready to cast off. Sue and I decided we would be the ones aboard the raft and the others would stay close to the shore for several reasons. First, to be the lookouts for HEP staff because we knew our clandestine operation was something they would not have allowed us to attempt. The second reason was in case we actually found the bird and could somehow corral it back toward them. The third reason, which maybe should have been the first reason, was in case something happened to me.

Several of the guys helped me from the chair onto the ground near the bank of the estuary where I proceeded to slide down the embankment on my butt to the raft. Sue then helped pull me aboard, the seat of my pants caked with dirt, grass and sand.

Off we went! I manned the front of the raft, lying on my stomach with my arms in the water with the hope that perhaps I could somehow steer us. Sue had made a makeshift paddle out of a length of stick and she was going to power the boat. Being on the water was a wonderful experience and I mostly just dangled my arms in it along the way.

It was a fairly good plan in theory. It really was. Unfortunately, we couldn't really get very far with the make-shift oar, nor could we steer the boat at all. We went all around the estuary edges much like a drunk person walks a straight line, but we did not see the night heron anywhere. It was afternoon and it was, after all, a night heron. So we should not have been surprised we couldn't find it. In fact, we didn't see many birds at all. It was probably a good thing we didn't find our injured bird because halfway around the estuary, I asked Sue if she had thought about what we would actually do if we spotted the heron. She hadn't thought that far ahead either. Even if we could get the bird into the boat, its talons no doubt would puncture it and then we would be sunk, literally. We did not have a plan for that!

We laughed so hard when we realized he absurdity of it all.

It really felt much like a Lucy and Ethel adventure. No one involved in the mission was sure that staff would believe it was mostly my idea to get on an inflatable raft and float around in the estuary. Our good intentions had been negated by our short-sighted plan, but the fun we had and the laughter it brought made it all worthwhile.

A few weeks later, the estuary was the site of another much-needed laugh at my expense when I tried my hand at fishing.

It happened after I had taken an informal poll of the residents in my apartment building about things they did to help them cope. A couple of the guys liked to fish and said it helped them to relax and de-stress. We had all seen them fishing in the estuary where they sometimes sent a wave excitement along the shoreline when they would hook a fish that was larger than their lines would hold. One of the guys really wanted me to try it, though I had only fished once in my life and that was when I was 11 or 12 years old. That was an outing that resulted in my catching a puny sunfish and spending most of my time trying to get it off my hook so I could throw it back in the water.

I had never really been a fan of fishing, mostly because no one could ever convince me that the fish are not in considerable pain and distress when they are hooked. But I had been on a roll in terms of setting an example by trying new things, so I told them I would give it a whirl.

If nothing else, I am pretty sure that watching me attempt to cast a line from my power wheelchair provided enough laughs to de-stress everyone there. I used my power chair like a four-wheeler and when I look at the terrain around the apartment building there today, I am not sure how I got to the places I used to go. I had to get near the water to cast the line, but I couldn't get real close because the bank was too steep. So, armed with the rod and reel the fisherman put together just for me, I sat and attempted to cast my line.

It soon became apparent that I wouldn't have to worry about removing any hooks from the mouths of any distressed fish because I rarely even got the line to the water's edge. Instead, my hook found every branch and clump of weeds in my general vicinity.

But I continued to cast as long as my fishing buddies would unsnag my line for me. Believe it or not, between the laughter at my lack of skill, the repetitive action and concentration I exerted to release the line at precisely the right time, it actually was an excellent coping exercise. Actually, it seemed to work pretty well for all of us, and clearly posed no threat to the fish.

    I still have that rod and reel.

13

Another mostly positive event that summer—and there were precious few-- didn't happen anywhere near the estuary, rather it unfolded about four miles away at the county courthouse where I went to vote.

When I could – and it never came easy -- I was determined to make the most of my situation. I tried to stay connected to the world and current issues. It was a local election year and I wanted to just be a normal person and vote. It was the first time early voting was offered, so I decided to take advantage of it.

It was hard to take wheelchair transport when you didn't know how long you would be somewhere, so I decided to just be transported there and that I would make my own way back in my power wheelchair. It was impossible to guess how long the early voting lines would take and when you gave wheelchair transport your time of return and weren't ready when they got there, they would leave after 10 minutes.

When I was dropped off, I couldn't find a place to cross the street where there was sidewalk curbing to get to the courthouse. I wheeled around on the street following the sidewalk, and didn't see any way to get up onto the sidewalk anywhere. I had to be mistaken, but as I wheeled around in circles trying to find it, I couldn't. I asked a grounds worker where I might find a wheelchair accessible entrance and he pointed to the back of the building.

He said, "Go back there to the dumpsters and hang a left.

Keep going and you'll see the ramp." I thought, wow, right behind the dumpsters was exactly where I was going to look next. I was surprised that there was absolutely no curbing anywhere on the courthouse side of the street where I was. I could have gone all the way back to the main street toward the eastern side of the building to get up on the sidewalk, but I would have to do that on the main road. I felt sure there had to be something around the front entrance side. I guess there really wasn't. I went back through the service entrance driveway, to the dumpsters and hung that left. I went in and got in line to vote early.

 I began to chit-chat with the ambulatory people around me in line about various things and mentioned about going to the dumpsters to get inside. They were pretty funny folks all around me and they seemed to enjoy my storytelling. I was sharing all of the backwards things I had encountered since being in a wheelchair. While I didn't find a lot of the experiences I had so far in the chair to be amusing, I was able to make light of them at that moment in the voting line. I wanted them to see me as me—an educated, funny and insightful woman. I didn't want them to get distracted or uncomfortable because of the wheelchair.

 Shortly afterwards, a gentleman approached me in this long line of people to ask if I would like to have a pamphlet about the issues that were up for a vote. He spoke slowly and loudly, and quite frankly, he was just a bit condescending. I thanked him anyway, and shared that I had educated myself on the candidates and amendment issues that were on the ballot. The people around me started asking why he only came to ask me if I wanted the pamphlet and a couple of them were incensed about it. They needed the brochure. Why did he talk like that to you, they asked?

 I chuckled, said I didn't know, but shared that often people in public places will talk to me slower and more loudly as if I am "slow" or hard of hearing. I tried to act as if this sort of thing didn't bother me, so that they would let it go as well. The truth was it did bother me. It bothered me a lot, and it was people like that guy who made me never want to be out in public. I couldn't be normal out here in the world in this chair. No one could see me anymore.

Three of the people in line around me began to ask the guy, one by one, if they could have the information, which began our discussion about the issues that were at stake at the polls. This was helpful for me. While I was making light, my feelings were hurt and I was disheartened by the experience. I knew I was overly sensitive to my treatment in the chair, but here I had people who witnessed it and commented that my perception was accurate. Either way, now I could share with my new groupies what I knew about the issues we were all about to vote on.

We ended up in a discussion about stem cell research, and which candidates were for it and which ones were against it. I asked them to share their views before I shared my perspective about it, and was able to educate them, I think, on what it really means, how they do it, etc. They were happy to hear the information. They shared that they honestly were only basing what they knew on what their political party's opinion was on the issue.

As we talked, the line was progressing slowly to the voting area. I had this little circle around me all the way through the lobby hall of the courthouse. These folks were all from different backgrounds, socio-economic statuses and political affiliations, but they were all gathered around and listening to what I had to say about stem cell research and what I had researched about the other issues on the ballot. I felt like they saw me. I could be sure they were hearing me.

We waited a really long time, so it was fortunate that I was able to distract us from the wait. There was a medical emergency inside the office where the polls were, but most of us seemed unaware of the long period of time we waited. We could hear the folks closer to the office door complaining about the wait, but by this point, they were asking me a lot of questions about my illness and circumstances. I didn't mind sharing because by sharing whatever personal things I was sharing, I was educating them even more. I was helping to dispel the myths about so many things with this group of people. Not only did they see how people in wheelchairs were treated first hand, but they also learned about stem cell research and homelessness.

We had to get back into single file once we entered the doorway into the actual office area where the polling staff were matching IDs and voter registration cards. A polling staffer began to motion for the person behind me to come ahead to the counter to show ID. The gentleman behind me was one of the people engaged in conversation with me, so he almost made a scene about me being passed over. I could see what was happening—the polling staffer saw that a taller counter area was available next, but the one that was at the wheelchair level was not, so he waved the man behind me forward. Since no one shared this information aloud, I shared that I could hand my ID and registration up to the taller counter without a problem, thanked my protector behind me for advocating for me and went on up there. Those counters were pretty high, but I could toss up my driver license and voter registration just the same.

    I did need more room for the chair to get into a polling cubby, so I asked for the room with fewer booths. Again the protective man behind me was not going to go ahead of me. I assured him it was fine, and that I needed more room. I thought this was pretty awesome. I had just met these people a little over an hour before this. The people in line with me helped to balance out the ick I felt from the condescending man handing out information pamphlets.

    I am not sure what made the people around me in line so open to what I had to say, or what made them respond to me differently than the pamphlet guy. Perhaps it was my chit-chatting that accounted for the connection. I can never know for sure, but I was grateful for how they were with me. They treated me like a regular human being and that was rarely the case for me navigating the world in a wheelchair. They had also become my advocates in the short period of time of talking with me. Even though this experience included one negative interaction and four or five positive interactions, at that time, I focused on the negative one for quite a while afterwards.

    I was sensitive about being in the chair and a lot of that was because I felt like a sitting target. It was often a challenge to get through a room filled with people and furniture. I spent a great deal of time feeling trapped with no way out of a room, or feeling like I was always in the way because the chair took up a lot of room. I was pretty hyper-vigilant before I got sick, but as a walking person, I could position myself to see the entire room and be near the exit. In a chair, it was not quite as simple.

    I often wondered if I ever treated any one in a wheelchair the way the pamphlet man treated me. He probably had no idea he was patronizing and condescending and maybe he found me to be the least intimidating of the people in line to approach. Perhaps I too had done this unconsciously. I thought that all people in wheelchairs couldn't walk. I thought if you were in a wheelchair that you couldn't take care of yourself and had to have an aide help you. I don't have any idea why I thought these things, but I must have picked up those ideas somewhere. I do know I was less than patient with anyone who moved slow or got in my way before I became slower myself.

    In a grocery store or in a parking lot, I would silently grumble when I had to wait for a person walking the crosswalk with a walker or using the very slow carts in the store. I realized one day very shortly after the symptoms began that I was now that person. It took me forever to do anything requiring movement, but I was so proud when I could do it myself. I found myself apologizing often to those behind me in a line at the store or waving the cars to go ahead because I knew it would take me forever to cross the crosswalk to get into the store from the parking lot.

    Before my illness, I used to think that they should get someone else to do it for them if they couldn't do it any faster than that. Didn't they know they were slowing down my obsessive-compulsive need to get from point A to point B as fast and efficiently as possible?

14

    I didn't plan to see a message of hope in my painting. It was supposed to be a painting about the depths of the darkness that was swallowing me.

    The first thing I did was slap on my canvas the darkest paint I had. I put some splotches of white randomly in the black for stars. For foreground, I painted tall blades of grass as if I were lying there looking up through it. Painting the grass was tedious, so I opted to leave an opening in it, which left a meandering path into the ominous sky.

    Hours had passed as the painting evolved, so I put down my brush and went outside for smoke. When I returned and looked at what I had created, I noticed something, something unintended: the pathway bordered by the grass ushered my eyes straight to the brightest of the stars, a star that gave off a glow. It had never been my intention to paint a tunnel to the light. The message of hope it conveyed was not what I wanted at all. I had been wallowing in my inner darkness, and what I saw made me angry. I felt dark, dammit, and now the painting took my eyes straight to a bright light, a beacon trying to lead me out of my darkness and despair.

    It wasn't the first time I received a message from an unlikely source, nor would it be the last. When I let go of the absurdity of being angry at a painting, I ended up embracing what it was telling me, and the hope it whispered to me could not have come at a better time.

I was no artist but had tried my hand at painting to help me cope and de-stress. I did it at the urging of a couple of my neighbors, who like everyone there were worried about the depth of my unhappiness.

It was November, approaching my four-month anniversary in the homeless project, and despite a few happy occasions, my depression had shrouded me in darkness, even to the point of taunting God and death.

I would run errands in my power chair several miles away on routes that included major intersections and found myself not caring if I got hit, secretly playing chicken with the traffic. In thunderstorms, I would sit in the parking lot and dare God to zap me with a bolt to lightning. I was a cauldron of anger and frustration. Struggling to get into the power chair each morning was my daily reminder how little control I had over anything.

Journal entry for 11/22/2004

It has been a while since I have sat here to write. Painful to do so with arms and hands. In meantime had to make painful decision to stop working my 12 hours at Directions. They tell me I can come back when I am ready. Still waiting on disability and also finally saw Dr. Frank last Friday to get an increase in baclofen. Insurance fiasco. Hoping the increase in baclofen will help the pain levels soon. Pain levels at a 7+ most always and 8+ with working. Does not seem that different but is some better the less I try to do.

Got to see the boys yesterday—such sweet creatures that have run away with my heart so strongly. Miss them always when not with them. Haven't missed a partner ever this much when absent. Reality of illness and level of dysfunction is scary to me. Not knowing so many things with that fear, though, I am allowing more creativity with my brain. Am limited to my expressions of such but am trying to do things that don't require fine motor skills. Next Tuesday makes four complete months I have been at Everybody's Tabernacle HEP—over it and ready to go. Tired of waiting/wondering. Figure there is reason enough for it and some deeper message. Always is. Have learned I can expand my interests here already and that given this set of circumstances, I am better at adapting than I once thought. Have so many things on my mind that I don't know what they even are anymore. Tearful more often than ever the past two months. Reality of the many losses I've incurred in under two years seems to be coming. I haven't begun to grieve them. Perhaps intermittently, but not totally. Scares me stupid to even imagine it all at once.

My physical pain was often unbearable, but the constant heartache I felt about not having my dogs with me was taking an equal, if not greater, toll.

Living without my dogs never got easier. There was nothing anyone could say or do to make me feel better about missing them. It seemed my visits with them only increased my pain, as if exponentially.

I carried around pictures of them, told everyone about them, and could be found staring at those images often. I imagined being a dog sandwich in my old bed at the house in Safety Harbor. I tried to not think of them, not miss them and to work on figuring out better ways of managing the pain and better ways of dealing with being without them. I would befriend anyone I would see with a dog, which only made me long even more to hold them in my arms.

The closest thing to a stand-in for my dogs was Sammy, a yellow lab mix that belonged to a HEP client named Wayne. In his mid-50s, Wayne was a recovering alcoholic and in remission from cancer when I knew him. He had been there so long and helped out so much, he had his own place and was allowed to have a dog, which was unheard of there. Sammy was a bit small for a lab but acted very much like one. I was so excited to meet her and she was equally excited to meet me. It was as if she knew I needed some lab kisses because she always gave me some. I was allowed to hog the time with Sammy when she was around because everyone knew I was lost without my boys.

Wayne would walk her over to the apartments in the mornings and in the evenings. The timing was usually perfect as we would have just fed, or were getting ready to a mass of mallards who always knew when it was feeding time. He would let her off leash in the field that was just to the south of the apartments and Sammy made a beeline toward us. She would sometimes run right into the water of the estuary if it was low tide.

 She would jump up on me, put her front paws on my lap, and kiss my face when she saw me. I looked forward to my visits with Sammy more than anyone could have known at the time. I felt better just being able to pet and give love to some being that was giving me only love back. I understand why the research shows that there is so much benefit from pet therapy—lower blood pressure, better immune functioning, reduced anxiety, and improved mood just to name a few. I didn't even feel as much pain when Sammy was around or when I was visiting the boys during this time. These times were opportunities for me to be in the moment without so much focus on the reality of my situation.

 But as much as I loved my time with Sammy, she always left me longing for my own boys who were always in my heart and on my mind. Not having them near was a constant reminder that I was still living in a homeless project, while the symptoms of my still unnamed disease were multiplying. I was becoming less able to take care of myself and that left me imagining that I would never be back living with my dogs again.

 These thoughts took me to very dark places, places where it no longer mattered if I had ALS because if I couldn't put my heart back together, then I didn't really care if I lived or died. But deep down I knew I had to keep caring, because if I gave up on myself I would also be giving up on my dogs and the promises I made to them. So, as much as I hated not being with them, it was because of their absence that I was driven to somehow, some way find my way back to them.

 I don't remember the details or the duration of my darkest times, probably for much the same reason I choose not to remember being without my dogs. I did pretty well some parts of some days, but most of the time I was steeped in darkness, a darkness that was always cruelest at night, especially nights when I was in pain, or my sleep medication didn't work. It was a darkness far worse than any darkness I had ever experienced, so much more was wrong, so much more was lost.

I needed to find something to help me cope. I still found peace in the birds and the ducks and watching the blue herons so exquisitely stalk their breakfast in the shallows, but more and more I was taking the estuary for granted. It was true that the estuary had given me the gift of stillness but my mind was unable to catch up to the stillness of my body.

It was clear that time by the estuary and being the go-to therapist were no longer enough to divert my thoughts from what was happening to my body and what had already happened to my life. Before I got sick, my coping skills were mostly physical. I would go shoot hoops or take a long run to manage my stress. My other coping skill was a pen and pad of paper. I would write and write as fast as I could until I felt better, an option now ruled out by the tremor in my right hand that made writing as impossible as going for a run.

It was that same tremor in my hand that at first made me balk at the suggestion of a neighbor that I try painting. If I was going to try something, I reasoned, it wasn't going to be something I was certain would only bring me more disappointment and frustration.

The neighbor who first suggested I try painting was a guy named Tom, who was one of my former clients when I was an outreach therapist. He was joined by my roommate, Sue, and another neighbor Linda in a campaign to get me to try it. Tom even brought me a paint-by-numbers set to get started. Despite my repeated arguments why I wouldn't be able to do it, they remained persistent. Finally, I got tired of hearing my own excuses and gave in.

I started with an etching tool because I simply could not stay within someone else's lines to paint by numbers. I decided to try to make a ceramic pot prettier using the etcher, which was an electric tool that fit in the palm of my hand. There were different sized tips for it to make different sized etchings into different materials. In truth, my secret intention was to prove to Tom, Linda and Sherry that this sort of thing was only going to frustrate me more, not help me cope. It turns out that even with the tremor, I could make some pretty cool stuff. I had to wear my wrist brace and make sure that my arm had something solid to rest upon and allow the tool to do the work.

I had no idea that I would be more fully learning a very important lesson about life in the process. I etched whatever the thrift store was throwing out, but soon moved on to painting with acrylics and bought some small canvases, brushes and paints. I was intrigued and entertained by the mixing of the colors to make new colors and variations of colors. I actually looked forward to painting.

What I learned was that I could paint fairly well if I didn't grip the paintbrush or try to control it. When you release control of the brush, you can create something beautiful. I let the brush do the work. My right hand tremor is an intention tremor, so when the hand and fingers are more relaxed, there is no shaking. It made no sense to me that I could paint tiny blades of grass, but could not write legibly with a pen. There was something meditative about painting, and that really helped me through the next year of my life when writing wasn't an option. My new friends and neighbors at the apartment building would gather around me when I was sitting outside working on a new project. They seemed happy to see me happy and some of them even ventured out to try new hobbies and coping strategies themselves.

Yes, I had found something to help me cope, really more of a distraction from the persistence of the darkness. Painting couldn't help me sleep when the pain stabbed at me. It could not stop the intermittent choking episodes when I did sleep. It couldn't end the haunting thought that I would never again be able to live on my own with my dogs. It couldn't stop the sickening fear I harbored of having to die so young. Worrying about death at 33 with so many hopes and dreams incomplete probably kept me up as much or even more than the pain. In my mind's eye one night, all I could see was the darkness of night. There were some stars, but they were almost fully eclipsed by the darkness, like dim blubs behind frosted glass.

That was the wretched emotional state I was in the day I painted that black sky, the sprinkling of stars and the grass that formed the accidental path to the light.

After I realized how silly I had been to be angry at a painting for interrupting my dark groove, I understood clearly the painting's message. It was telling me that no matter how dark it feels for me, somewhere inside me there is still a spark of hope flickering that will see me through my nightmare.

It was nearly dawn when I had completed the painting, and I could hardly wait to share with someone how it had evolved in spite of myself. I decided I would present it to my counselor, Jenny, when I went for a session with her later that morning.

The paint wasn't even dry when I gave it to her in a frame with no glass. It was no masterpiece but the story behind it was a masterpiece of the epiphany.

15

    I never would have imagined that a message I got from a painting while in a terrible, dark place would be just what I needed to help keep me going. It was like a beam from a flashlight trying to show me the way to a purpose, assuring me it was out there even if I couldn't see it yet.

    It was also as though it tucked a bookmark into the pages of my story, marking a place for me to take a kind of break from everything that was tormenting me. I knew that whatever awaited me would be no less of a cruel obstacle course than I had already faced, but now there was something telling me not to give up. It was a turning point, I guess, but I had no idea where it would lead me. It did, however, prompt me to find some way to get out of the homeless project and into my own place again with my dogs. It also got me to stop putting off the things I would have to do to get there.

    Going to the county offices to apply for a health insurance plan, food stamps and other services to which I was entitled was something I had been putting off far too long. In the past I had spent untold hours there with my homeless clients advocating for them so they could get the same things I would now be trying to get for myself. The clients I helped there had been mostly street homeless who weren't treated like human beings, so I enjoyed going with them to help facilitate an understanding that whether they smell or look unkempt, they are, indeed, human and not that unlike the rest of us.

But this visit would be so different. This time I wasn't the therapist with the clients. This time I was a homeless woman in a wheelchair and I was on my own. The idea of having to sit there and wait, just as my clients used to wait, was not exactly appealing. I had already grown weary of advocating for myself, and was beginning to understand the apathy my clients encountered in those same situations.

Knowing I had put it off long enough, I decided to travel the three miles or so to the country offices in my power chair. I wanted to be there when it opened at 8 am, so I would have a better chance of getting what I needed without having to do it over two days, the same way I used to try to do it with my clients.

I didn't mind travelling in my chair. It was a risk to cross a main intersection, even with the walk signal, because motorists just don't see below their eye level. But, unlike other times, I was careful on this day. I got there with time to spare but my promptness did little to speed up the process. I signed in and proceeded to wait six hours before I was seen by a caseworker. The workers I knew, ones who had helped me with my clients in the past, walked by me at least twice—once on their way to lunch and once on the way back. The only time any of the other workers talked to me was when my power chair was in the way.

Finally, my name was called, and by a familiar face. Once she recognized me, she was in shock by my appearance and the wheelchair. The woman who had called me, and all the others who knew me, said, "Why didn't you tell us you were here? What has happened to you?!" I told them that they walked right past me twice and that I had even said hello. They said they didn't recognize me, which I decided was okay since I didn't recognize me anymore, either.

The truth is, I wasn't looking forward to having to explain why I looked so awful and the chair and the homelessness. I didn't go out of my way to seek them out, but had hoped they would see my name on the sign-in sheet and expedite things. We visited for a bit and I shared with them where I was living, and they all said to give them a call directly if I needed any other services. I was torn between being grateful that I knew people there and wishing I could just be invisible and anonymous through it all. I couldn't make up my mind whether to want to be invisible or to be seen and heard for who I was. Being acknowledged and being anonymous both seemed to be so hard anymore.

They said they weren't sure how they could handle living where their clients lived and all I could say was that there is great truth in the fact that homelessness could indeed happen to anyone of us. The process from there was a bit quicker and I applied for food stamps and got my county health plan card. As many times as I have said to others, "There is nothing wrong with getting the services you need because that is what they are there for," you would think that I would have had no issue at all getting them. I was certainly grateful that the services were there, regardless of my pride-related issues about needing them. My rational mind was telling me it is fine, you are eligible for all this, but the rest of my mind was reminding me it was simply more proof my life was out of control.

Nonetheless, I held close to a renewed inkling of hope, and counted my trip to the county office as a positive in that I got the things I had set out to get. But there was much more to it than that. It was a first step toward the next phase of my improbable journey, one that would get considerably worse before it got dramatically and wonderfully better.

16

There was a restlessness stirring in me, a longing that kept nudging me forward despite my pain, immobility and ongoing bouts of darkness.

It was now January, 2005, making it just over five months that I had lived at the homeless project. I had moved there in late July as a temporary measure, and it had already been much longer than my idea of temporary. I was determined to change my situation and do whatever it took for as long as it took to one day get my own place again. I wanted that for so many reasons. There was my burning desire to be reunited with my dogs, of course, but I also dreamed of being independent again with a sense of purpose that my illness was so relentlessly bent on taking from me.

My starting point included my food stamps, my county health plan and $837 a month in in Social Security disability insurance, which I had been approved for in December. But the choice I made for my next living arrangement would have less to do with money than rehabilitation and learning how to function day-to-day within my limitations.

My condition had deteriorated since my move to the homeless program. I was having trouble moving my arms above my shoulders because of muscle spasms and the muscles in my feet, calves, arms and hands were so tight it felt like they were turning a vice on my bones.

I don't recall who suggested a skilled nursing and

rehabilitation center, but I grew to love the idea, at least in theory. My thinking was that with some intensive physical and occupational therapy, I could improve my ability to do everyday things. I also reasoned that such a place could improve my strength since I would be getting three nutritious meals a day. I figured that after a few months they could better evaluate my level of mobility so that I could better determine if living on my own with my dogs was even a realistic possibility.

I was further encouraged when I discussed the idea with my neurologist who was supportive and said he would write the order I would need to get into such a place. So my mind was made up, although I should have known getting there would hardly be a cakewalk.

While the process was easier than filing for bankruptcy and Social Security disability, it was just about as unpleasant. Once the ball starts rolling, you have less than 30 days to be in a nursing/rehab facility full time. It started with a visit from a woman with the Department of Elder Affairs who asked me a slew of questions to help her gauge what I was able to do and what I wasn't able to do. She was sweet, compassionate and gave me as much information about the process as she knew. She wasn't used to evaluating people my age, especially one who asked as many questions as I did, but she handled it well.

If I didn't feel badly enough about my physical limitations, the evaluation served to make me feel worse. I had been pretending to do some of my activities for daily living for a while, but really, it was my roommate who completed all the household chores. It was another reality check when I saw my own answers in black and white on the evaluation papers. The conclusion was simple: the way I was trying to do things was not safe.

With my evaluation completed and with my neurologist's blessing, I set out to find a suitable facility. I began my search from a list the elder affairs worker had given me. The best ones on the list only accepted Medicare or private insurance. I couldn't afford private insurance and I would have to wait two years from the time I started getting Social Security until I would be eligible for Medicare benefits.

I was covered by the Medicaid Share of Cost program, which isn't true Medicaid. Here is how it worked: I had to spend 837 dollars and then the insurance covered the rest of the month. Once I meet the amount of medical costs, I will have the rest of my health care covered by the state. Where I was supposed to come up with the $837 was beyond me, but my prescriptions alone totaled twice that amount.

Anyway, the coverage I had left me with limited options for rehabilitation.

I have helped friends and family members find nursing homes before, so I knew what questions to ask and what to look for when visiting them. I felt confident I could make a good choice among the ones left. I started by selecting places that were either close to where my dogs were staying or close to my dad's house. I visited a couple of them but was turned down.

Their marketing people were gracious and I enjoyed meeting them, but they informed me I was too young and wouldn't fit in there. They said it would be in my best interest not to be there. I really didn't care that there would be no residents there my age, and I have always enjoyed being around seniors. I think it was more of a case of looking out for the best interests of the other residents and not mine. Either way, it was another disappointment, especially since both locations were ideal and both places would have accepted my insurance.

Being turned away like that also served to aggravate my already worsening pain levels and mobility. I was rapidly losing patience with the search process and the clock was ticking.

I ended up selecting a place based on a tree. Well, not solely on a tree, but the tree is what helped seal the deal. It was a beautiful, lone oak that stood in a grassy swale just below the driveway. It was perfectly shaped, its fullness and roundness billowing out evenly above and out from its trunk. It gave me a peaceful feeling.

It was the STH Nursing and Rehabilitation Center, located on a quiet street in Clearwater. I was assured it had everything I needed in terms of nutrition, rehabilitation and internet access. Its residents included a wide range of ages and disabilities. Oh, and the marketing representative said she often brings her little fluffy dog in to see the patients.

On the surface, things seemed to be falling into place. I made the decision to move there, made all the necessary arrangements, and assured everyone in my life that it would be a temporary move, benefit me greatly, and pave the way for me to live on my own again. It was a done deal, and the last Friday in February would be my last day living at the homeless project.

Leaving HEP was far less eventful than arriving, although I would miss the good parts of living there and many of the people there. Once the wheels of Elder Affairs start turning, it seems that everything happens very quickly, so I felt like my head was spinning around and I am not sure I was really feeling anything but numbness when it was time to go. While I was reassuring everyone that this was a positive move, I was also trying to reassure myself that I was making a decision that at least had more potential to get me back with my dogs than anything I had tried to make happen there.

There was a nice dose of hope bubbling in me the day I headed off to take the next twist in the road. I didn't know what was ahead, but I couldn't help feeling a sense of accomplishment. I got myself out of the homeless project with a plan I believed would begin to change the direction of my life.

I never thought that I could have been fooled by a tree.

17

    It was raining hard the Friday afternoon I arrived at the nursing home. A storm front had settled in the area the day before and was showing no signs of backing off. The ominous weather turned out to be the perfect escort for my entrance.

    What I dealt with that first weekend there left my head spinning, wondering how I could have ever picked such a place, and set the general tone for how my three-month stay there would go.

    I had been there less than six hours when a serious problem arose regarding my night medications. When the nurse brought them I discovered an important pill wasn't among them. The missing pill was a higher dose of a drug my neurologist had put me on to see if it would help with my increasing spasticity. It wasn't a drug I could just stop taking without consequences. Not having it meant I would spend the weekend withdrawing from it, which meant more pain and spasticity. I would have to start all over with the lowest dose of the same drug Monday once they reached my doctor. Apparently, the admitting doctor who was contracted by the facility missed this medication on my medication list. Granted, there were more than a dozen medications on that list, but each had a purpose.

    The next issue related to the portable elevated potty chair that I need so I can use the toilet safely. The bathroom I was to use was between two bedrooms. There were two patients per bedroom, so our bathroom would be shared by four people. I explained to an aide who helped me get settled that the armed potty chair would always have to be left over the toilet so that I could transfer to it from my wheelchair. She said that wouldn't be a problem.

As it turned out, it would be a problem.

I needed to use the bathroom when I awoke in the middle of the night from a restless, pain-interrupted sleep. When I got to the bathroom the potty chair was not over the toilet where I was assured it would be. It was in the bathroom all right, but nowhere near the toilet. I couldn't find anyone down the hall at the nurses' station to help, so I moved it myself the best I could from my wheelchair. I wasn't able to get it exactly how it was supposed to be placed and was just lucky I didn't hurt myself when I used it. My bathroom trip was made even more treacherous since the floor was sopping wet from a streaming leak in the ceiling from the ongoing rain.

And there were still a couple more surprises left in my first-night treat bag.

Not long after my bathroom episode, I was lying in my bed trying to fall asleep when I was jarred awake by a woman's shrill, panicked screams. She sounded like she was freaking out in the bathroom. I found out later she was a dementia patient from the adjacent room who apparently became distraught when she encountered my elevated potty chair.

The third act of my potty chair drama came about 6 a.m. when I was informed by the nursing staff that I would have to place the portable potty beside my bed and keep it there for the duration of my stay. Imagine my delight in hearing that. Did I really have to use the potty chair next to my bed because the real bathroom wasn't accessible for me? Despite my protests, the decision stood and I was stuck with the potty chair beside my bed. I was horrified that I would have to use it there where I would have no privacy. They assured me it would be emptied regularly.

So much had gone wrong, and I had only been there about 12 hours. At least I wasn't caught off guard when things didn't improve on my second day, starting with my morning medications.

I was taking 12 different drugs. Some I took three or four times a day, others as needed. I looked into the medication cup and they were wrong again. I showed the nurse my medication sheet and showed her which medication she forgot to include in my cup. The nurses weren't big fans of being corrected, and while they were apologetic, they weren't eager to see me coming toward them in those early days.

Then there was the matter of food, or rather the lack of it. My meager breakfast of some sort of egg product and one stale piece of toast, looked similar to a sparse dinner plate they gave me the night before. It appeared they had me on a calorie-restricted diet instead of one that would facilitate weight gain to help me build strength. In fairness, I hadn't met with the dietary staff yet so my menu would be something else I hoped I rectify on Monday.

By mid-morning Saturday, rain was still lashing my bedroom window, I was in pain, sleep deprived, and hungry. I was experiencing withdrawal from medication I had missed, which meant a marked increase in my pain and spasticity. I believe there were only two doses of medication that were correct all weekend. I remember having a mounting feeling of concern for the well-being of other patients there whose mental capacities were diminished. They didn't even know what medications they were taking, let alone whether what they got was right.

The rain never really let up that weekend, and by Sunday morning there were several plastic buckets on the bathroom floor that were close to overflowing. There were also several rain-soaked chunks of fallen ceiling tiles on the floor.

Finally, shortly before noon Sunday, something happened that perked me up a bit.

The place got a surprise visit from the Florida's Agency for Health Care Administration (AHCA), the state regulating body for all such facilities. When they approached me to talk about how things had been going, they wouldn't have to worry about lulls in the conversation.

I had plenty to say about what I had already observed in the two days I had been there. It wasn't all just about how I had been treated. I also commented on deficiencies I noticed in everything from patient care to staffing levels. I appreciated being able to tell someone who might be able to make some changes. I felt a little like that undercover reporter I once had wanted to be, exposing the shady facility. I was told that anything I told them would be confidential. The funny thing about confidentiality is that it really only means that my name wouldn't be used, but with the comments I offered, it wouldn't take a genius to know it was me.

There had been many other times in my life when a situation presented itself as a worthy cause. The downside of my good intentions is that they usually end up making matters worse for me. I would learn soon enough that this would be another one of those times, but I have never been easily deterred when I see wrongs that need to be righted.

I was about to embark on a personal crusade to fix this nursing home, a decision that was hastened when I found out from the AHCA agent who interviewed me that I would have to stay there at least 30 days before I could go anywhere else. If I had my way, I would have been looking for another nursing home first thing Monday morning, but since I was stuck there I was determined to put my time to good use. This would be a perfect opportunity for me to do what I do best—advocate for those who can't advocate for themselves. I have always loved advocating for others and because of my illness I had gotten better at advocating for myself. This would be a chance to do both.

So when Monday arrived I had quite a list to discuss with anyone who would listen. I found out I would have to take my complaints to the director of nursing. At our first encounter she seemed happy to meet with me about my concerns, but during the month that followed, it became apparent that her patience was growing thin as was her enthusiasm for my frequent visits. I was relentless because it was impossible for me to ignore what was happening around me and with my own care. Whether she liked it or not, I simply couldn't help myself.

Somewhere about my third week there, I did begin to

temper what I reported and what I didn't, but continued to air concerns throughout my stay. They weren't used to dealing with a patient as perceptive and vocal as me, and certainly not someone with my background.

Having managed group homes for the chronically mentally ill and worked in homeless shelters where medications were locked up and monitored by staff, I was aware of the need for medication policies and safeguards. I had developed such policies and procedures in the past. To my surprise (or horror), there were no such systems at this place.

The shortcomings were hardly limited to medications safeguards. Problems were rampant, encompassing everything from hygiene practices and staff shortages. There were so many things wrong that by my third week, I had some patients poised to start a coup. But that idea was quelled when it became clear that far more patients were just not willing to get involved, particularly the ones whose situations meant this facility was the only home they had. While they agreed medication errors were bad and that the general quality of care wasn't good, they just didn't want to risk being seen as trouble makers. It didn't really matter to them that other non-ambulatory patients, myself included, could only get two showers a week because we needed help transferring and bathing. That could only improve with a staff increase. While the other patients empathized, they felt it really wasn't their cause since they could take a shower on their own whenever they wanted.

I had been there just over a month and my nursing home rehab plan was turning out to be everything I didn't want it be. The good news was that despite the lousy treatment I was getting and would continue to get for the rest of my time there, I would discover a way to help myself. I also refused to resign myself to the idea of being stuck in a place like that and was able to keep alive my dream of getting back into a place of my own with my dogs.

Something else happened late in my second month there, something encouraging related to treatment of my illness, something that had nothing to do with the nursing home. My neurologist had me undergo a trial in which baclofen – the drug that relaxes my muscles to ease spasticity -- was injected directly into my spinal canal. I learned it was possible to have a pump implanted to provide a constant flow of the drug into my spine. A representative from the pump company evaluated changes in my spasticity levels during the four-hour trial period and determined that delivering the drug in that way would work much better, far surpassing what happens when I take the drug orally.

But I didn't even know what I had or whether I would ever be a candidate to have such a pump implanted. I did know such an operation would be expensive and I wouldn't even be able to consider it for 18 months when I would qualify for Medicare. There would be hope then, but it wasn't going to help me now.

Still, I did tuck it away in the back of my mind where I still kept secret dreams. I didn't know then that the test would foreshadow a change that would come as dramatically and unexpectedly as the illness had struck me.

But for now, all I knew for sure was that I was in a nightmare of a nursing home and needed to find my way out.

18

The room where they held physical therapy sessions had drab, pale green walls. The floor was covered by a worn grey carpet. The physical therapist in charge sat at a desk near the door and the speech therapist sat at the opposite side of the same wall. In the far corner, there was a mock bed with a rail, a machine that stood you upright, and some weight equipment. The walls were mostly blank with the front that abuts the hallway all windows.

I remember so much about that room because during my weekly, hour-long therapy sessions, I was just left there, sitting in my wheelchair. I had a lot of time to look around. Oh, they had given me some arm exercises to do, but they were utterly impossible. I was supposed to do use the resistance band and pull and push and such, but my arms really couldn't pull that band at all without them feeling like they were shaking off my body. It didn't seem to matter to anyone that I couldn't do it, and I was convinced the director of physical therapy prescribed that exercise just to spite me.

So I would sit there the entire time making futile attempts at the arm curls while watching the physical therapy assistant help other patients. No one came over to me. I had no one to tell that I couldn't do the exercise or to show what was happening when I tried.

But the more I sat there, the more I became intrigued by what they were teaching the others. They were learning how to transfer safely from their wheelchairs to pretend beds that looked much like a mattress sample you might see at the mattress stores, and other maneuvers to help them with daily living. They showed them the proper ways to transfer both with a board and directly using a leg or whatever the patient had that worked. They were also being shown how to use specialty gadgets designed to help them do things from their wheelchairs. There was one that was a reaching/grabber tool. You squeezed the trigger and it grabbed things fairly well that were far away. I became much more than a curious observer. I was in full watch-and-learn mode.

I hadn't been at the place for long when I came to a critical realization: these people were not going to help me get better at doing anything. That notion actually worked in my favor, since I vowed that what they weren't going to teach me to do, I would teach myself. I reasoned that if I could figure out ways to do things there that I wasn't supposed to be able to do, I could do them living on my own.

The first indication that they were not going take my strength and rehabilitation plan seriously came the first week when a staff social worker came to my room to have me sign my treatment plan. The plan was all written out for me and had been approved by others who had already signed it. I was stunned to learn they had a treatment team meeting about me and I wasn't invited.

I know about treatment planning—I had been doing treatment plans with clients since 1992. It is considered best practice to involve patients in the process because it allows them to have input and be more invested. I was interested in why some of the things were on my plan and told them I wanted to be part of the process. Maybe they weren't used to that sort of thing or maybe other higher functioning patients didn't care much about their treatment plans, but I really didn't care about their thought processes. I had put myself in this awful place, and was damn sure going to get something for my trouble. I started attending my treatment team meetings where they succeeded in making me feel like I was imposing. All I was trying to do was clarify my symptoms, share what I thought I needed help with in physical therapy, and identify my personal treatment goals. I thought it was important that they knew what I hoped to achieve. Instead, it appeared they had decided that because my chart still said "Rule out ALS" it meant I probably had ALS, and they didn't see a point to try to do much. They were also acting as if I was going to be there indefinitely, which was the furthest thing from my mind.

Their original treatment plan for me was focused on my lower body only. That would have been fine except that my inability to do daily tasks – bathing most notably -- was created by my arms. The wheelchair worked as my legs, but I really needed my arms to be able to do things from the chair. I also shared that I would like to learn how to better do tasks from the chair.

Those impossible arm exercises and being left to fend for myself in the therapy room were my reward for getting involved. After the first treatment plan meeting I attended, that same director of physical therapy who saddled me with those exercises, never once made eye contact with me right up to and including the day I was discharged.

If I felt as if I had entered the twilight zone when I moved into the homeless project, here I felt like I had followed Alice down the rabbit hole and fallen helplessly into a place where nothing made sense, where up was down and down was up. It was a place where no one seemed to see me, though I knew I was there, and no one seemed to hear me, though I knew I was speaking.

If I was ever going to find the door out of there, I would have to find it by myself.

To do it meant I would have to be my own physical therapist. I would have to practice doing things myself. But before I did anything I had to stop wasting time and energy being incensed over not getting what I needed. It took a few weeks for the anger to seep out of me but as it did, I was learning to work with my symptoms rather than fight them.

I didn't have to go far to start working on my own. The potty chair right beside my bed presented a formidable challenge that took some practice and all my strength to overcome. I not only hated that potty chair because of where they made me put it, I hated it because it didn't have an arm rest that would drop down to make it easier for me to safely slide onto it from my bed. Instead, I had to simultaneously grab its fixed arms and pull myself into a position to twist and plunk myself into the seat. It was disheartening. There was trial and error, my arms trembling under the strain of steadying myself. But my resolve triumphed. I figured out how to do it, an accomplishment that gave me renewed hope that I would also be able to do it living on my own.

  Gradually I found myself doing more on my own than I even thought possible. I started paying attention to those things so that I could try them out in a different environment. I practiced some household chores at Dan's when I visited my dogs and figured out how to use the bathroom there safely. I vacuumed and dusted. I also tried out cooking on his stove as it was far more accessible that the one in the kitchen on my apartment at HEP. My only concern was bathing. I still couldn't do that without the right assistive equipment or help from someone to transfer to the shower bench.

  By now I had been there about seven weeks, had stopped attending my treatment team meetings, and had backed off my weekly complaint sessions with the director of nursing. I had turned inward to find a way out. I was beginning to envision myself reunited with my dogs and living on my own again. I was overcoming some physical obstacles, making progress with some daily living tasks. I was beginning to see that if I could figure all of this out in different environments, then with the right assistive equipment, I could probably figure out how to do it on my own. I also started going outside more often to listen to stories and let the remnants of my anger dissipate in swirls of cigarette smoke.

  The nursing home didn't have an estuary with blue herons and ducks, but there were lots of birds and squirrels to feed and no shortage of smokers. I hadn't lost my love of a good story.

  The stories I loved best were told by an attractive, older Italian man who claimed to have ties to the mafia. He was living there because his heart only worked at 20 percent capacity and could stop at any time. I would ask him to tell me a story and he would always oblige me. We became friends and his presence there made my stay a bit easier. We would sit and smoke and exchange tales, me telling him one about my dogs, him telling me one about the mob. I don't know if his stories were true but it didn't really matter. They were action-packed dramas with plenty of humor. They sounded like episodes from "The Sopranos" and distracted me from the bleak stories that keep running through my head, stories about me never getting my dogs back or having to live in some kind of assistive facility for the rest of my life.

I tried to talk with him as much as I could because there were so many others there whose voices were steeped in resignation and helplessness. Sometimes as I listened, I found myself combatting my own doubts and fears that I might end up just like them—stuck and not giving a damn.

There was one person my age who had cancer. He was in another remission, but had no interest in ever leaving the place for a less restrictive assisted living facility. He had been in remission before and the cancer came back, so for him it was easier to stay put rather than jump through the bureaucratic hoops it would take for him to leave only to have the cancer return. He just seemed so sad. His legs were too weak to walk far, so he rode a small scooter. His perspective made it seem he was already dead.

Another person I sometimes talked with had suffered a stroke and had lost the use of the left side of his body. He told me he had given up on physical therapy. I encouraged him to work with the physical therapists and told him about research that showed the brain has the ability to work around damage and learn to do things in a different way. At times, I wasn't sure who I was trying to convince, him or me.

You see, I could relate to the resignation, since I had felt its tug before. I just couldn't fall victim to it this time for fear I would never get out of there. The sadness and defeat in their voices were not unlike what I heard so many times before in the voices of my homeless clients. It occurred to me that many of the long-term nursing home patients were essentially homeless themselves. Whatever they might have had before having to go into the nursing home, they no longer had.

Whatever I once had was also gone. My illness had seen to

that. It had brought me to homelessness. It had brought me to a nursing home. It had tried to sink me in my own darkness. The despair I was seeing in others was tempting me. But I had forces away from the nursing home that kept me moving forward, my dogs first and foremost among them.

While at the nursing home, I was only allowed to make day trips to see Duke and Amore about once every two weeks. I would get dropped off at Dan's house about 8 in the morning and stay until the wheelchair transport van would make its last run to the nursing home about 7 in the evening. I sucked up every ounce of love my dogs could give. More than anyone or anything else, they kept me from giving in to the resignation and apathy that stalked me. Their faces, their eyes, their love were my greatest motivators. They were the transfusion my spirit needed. They reassured me, reminded me of the promises I made to them, and rejuvenated my resolve to get the three of us back together in our own place. I cried every single time our visit was over.

I was also motivated by family and friends who I missed, but had also forbidden to visit me there. I let my dad bring me lunch a few times, but I would always meet him in the court yard. I wouldn't allow him or anyone else to come inside. They already had etched in their minds the terrible image of what my illness had done to me, and I didn't want to have them add to that the sight of me in a place like this. I could barely stand it myself, and wasn't about to invite them in for a close-up look.

I kept contact with them on the Internet, made available to me by a kind social worker who let me use her computer when she could. But as my days there dragged on and my access to the computer became sporadic, I was feeling increasingly disconnected from everyone. When I was able to touch base with them, I reassured them I would be out of here in no time and see them and talk to them soon. As I typed those messages, I was also sending a message to myself: even if ALS wasn't ruled out, this was not going to be the last place I would live.

If it wasn't going to be the last place I would live, it would most assuredly be the most absurd. Sometimes the absurdity crossed over to hilarity, like the morning Goldilocks – more accurately Silverlocks--paid a visit.

I had gotten up early for a medical test and gone out for a coffee and cigarette. When I wheeled back into my room, there was a woman with snow-white hair sleeping in my bed. Her eyes were closed and her mouth was opened to form a perfect O. Her wispy hair fell back on the pillow as if she had placed it there meticulously to not touch her face and forehead. She was the same dementia patient who had freaked out my first night there over my potty chair being in the bathroom. She looked like a corpse, and I was horrified to think she had just walked in to my room, lied on my bed and died. She certainly appeared to have a death grip on one of my stuffed animals – a black dog – which she clutched across her chest.

I went and got an aide who, to my relief, discovered my visitor wasn't dead. In fact, she was very much alive, protesting loudly and vehemently when the aide stirred her awake and tried to get her out of my bed. She was talking but making no discernible sense. She clearly had no idea where she was, grabbed my blanket and the stuffed dog, and snuggled back up onto my pillow. While it made for good entertainment for 5:30 a.m., I had to use the potty chair next to my bed. I wouldn't be able to do that for another 45 minutes because that's how long it took the aides to calm her down enough to get her up and back to her own room.

Another morning I awoke at 4 am to see the aides taking clothes out of my closet to put on my roommate. She weighed about 200 pounds, was fed through a feeding tube, and couldn't speak or do much of anything except maybe bite an occasional aide. I probably weighed maybe 110 and my clothes obviously were never going to fit a woman her size. I lay there in my bed watching the two aides trying to tug my sweatpants onto her body, shaking my head and wondering what in the world they could be thinking. Did they think my sweats were going to magically expand to fit? But it was amusing, so I let them try for a while before telling them they had the wrong patient's clothes. My rotund roommate was never happy to have an aide help her do anything, and although she couldn't really speak, she could scream and screech like a blue jay. This time I couldn't blame her.

It was funny or it was sad, but whatever you prefer, I had seen and heard enough of it. I wanted out more than those aides wanted those pants to fit, and more than Silverlocks didn't want to get up.

19

    One of my dogs was about to lead me toward a brave new turn in my improbable journey. It may not be easy to understand how it happened, except to trust in the indescribable connection I have always had with Duke, the smaller of the two, the one who first got up and came to me at the shelter the day I adopted them.
    Duke and I seem to have always been able to communicate by eye contact alone, and there was something different in his eyes during a visit soon after I had vowed to get out of that place. Duke sat in front of me, pawing me until I took his paw and met his eyes. But this was much more than his usual greeting. This time there was an urgency in his stare. He fixed his soulful eyes on mine for what seemed like five minutes. His gaze was relentless and I was experiencing a flood of emotions. I found myself in tears, telling him that I didn't know how to make things different. I would try to avert my eyes, but he kept making me return to his gaze. His eyes were pleading, and it was clear to me what he wanted. He was telling me to get us back together, that he was trusting me to do that.
    His message couldn't have been clearer if he had emailed it. I left there that day knowing it was time. I had absolutely no idea how to make it happen, but I was definitely going to figure it out. It was time to be living under the same roof with my dogs.
    The next day was Sunday, so I bought a newspaper out of the box at the front entrance of the nursing facility, and started looking for a place. I am not sure I cared where it was if it was close to dad or Dan or Karen. I called about them in all of those areas.
    I left a lot of messages and when I got call backs I found out

the places had been rented. I got the same results when I didn't hear back and made follow up calls. The unsuccessful phone campaign was made further unpleasant since I had to use the phone in my room where the smell or urine was a regrettable constant. When I did reach someone, I found out they didn't want my large dogs there or that the place wasn't wheelchair accessible. I was discouraged, but I knew there had to be a way.

    I needed first to find an alternative to the phone in my room where my overweight roommate's condition was an added distraction. I took my power chair to a Target a few miles away where I bought a prepaid cell phone. Now I could actually get the return calls. Several places allowed dogs, but weren't wheelchair accessible. Another problem was that places that sounded promising were rented before I could schedule a wheelchair transport ride to look at them. I had to arrange my transportation a day ahead and a lot of the apartments were being rented the same day they were advertised.

    After a couple of weeks of this, I was beginning to lose faith, but it only took another visit with my dogs to recharge my battery and push me forward.

    I was also bolstered by some of my nursing home friends who encouraged me and brainstormed with me about how I might overcome potential living problems once I get into a place. I would be challenged in just about area of daily living, from bathing to cooking to cleaning. Safety was my first priority. Bathing was my biggest concern going into this adventure but I felt certain I could do it at least twice a week, which would be more than what I often received there. I just had to figure out the rest. My Italian friend was the most helpful and rational. He asked me questions and posed scenarios I would not have considered without his input. Some were issues he was unable to find solutions to for himself and the reason he was still there.

    A new plan was beginning to form. I was going to make this happen and it seemed I went overnight from waning hope to having more resolve than I had had since my illness had begun. It was time and that is all I knew.

I started asking more questions about the process of getting out of there. I still didn't know where I would go, but wanted to know how long I needed to plan ahead with SSDI, Medicaid and the Elder Affairs powers that be. I really did my homework for the discharge. I not only talked to the facility's social worker, but asked and researched from other sources, including Social Security itself. I even got help from the physical therapy assistant who used to ignore me. Since she knew my time there was ending she started to show me a few things that would be helpful, things I had seen her teach other residents. I would be leaving the nursing home at the end of May, provided I could find a place for the dogs and me by that time.

There were skeptics of my newly developing plan. Some were friends and family from the outside and others were professionals and friends from the inside. Each time someone would share their specific reasons for their skepticism, I would offer solutions to their issues. I had back up plans for everything I might encounter. If I had the right assistive equipment, I was certain I could somehow figure out how to make this happen. My brother would help me get the equipment I would need once I found a place.

20

The unit I found was a duplex and really a bit of a dump. It had a fenced-in yard, private from the adjoining duplex and my dogs were welcome without any additional pet deposits. It was in Dunedin and the rent was right. I called the landlord, and he had just met with someone he could have rented it to. I explained about wheelchair transport and asked if he would be willing to please wait until I could at least see it. He agreed. I scheduled wheelchair transport and went there the following day.

I couldn't get all the way inside in my chair, but immediately saw ways that we could remedy that. The doorframes would have to be removed so that my chair could get through the inside doors, and ramps were needed for both the front and back doors. My landlord physically picked me up from my chair and carried me through the apartment so I could see what the bathroom looked like to figure out how to make it accessible for me. He was okay with the modifications that were going to be needed.

He rented it to me and brought a lease back for me to sign at the nursing home the next day. It was going to be another few weeks before I would be able to move in because of the nursing home entrapment and that would be perfect because it might take that long to do the modifications. I was going to need that time to find someone to cheaply build me ramps, tear out the doorframes, and for my brother to help me to pay for and order the special assistive equipment I was going to need to be on my own. My brother was awesome and let me get whatever I thought I might need, so I ordered everything I had seen the Medicare patients using in the physical therapy room. I still had my mattress and bookshelves in storage, along with a television and a few things I kept from my former life. I got the phone numbers of a couple of the nurse's aides I liked and made a deal with myself that I would call them if I was unable to keep up with personal hygiene things with the assistive equipment in place.

I hadn't been so excited about something in a long time. I had about 20 days before I could escape the nursing home, and during the interim, I made several visits to my future home. I was getting things ready, brainstorming mobility challenges, and just picturing my new life. I was going to make it work.

On what would be my last visit to see my dogs at Dan's, I practiced walking them alongside me in the power chair. I had been watching "The Dog Whisperer" on my weekend visits for months, and I could almost visualize us being able to walk together. This was important to me because I felt that they deserved to get to do the things that dogs get to do. They had already been through so much in their young life and I was determined to make the rest of it as stable and happy as I could possibly make it. Our first walk was not that great, but I saw that it was definitely going to be possible with some practice. I could give them a good life and take care of myself enough along the way. We were really going to do this.

I gathered up folks to take me to storage and to get some things I would need. My brother, dad, sister-in-law and step mom helped to clean the place before moving day. They helped to get things ready the week before it would be my break out of the nursing home.

It was May 28, 2005 and I was finishing off my time at the nursing home. I had to wait until the month ended to be able to get my disability income sent directly back to me instead of the nursing home. The arrangement while I was in the nursing home was they would get all but $20 of my monthly income. The nursing home would then give me that 20 dollars as spending money. I was so close to getting out of there, getting back with my dogs, and the time couldn't pass quickly enough.

A handyman friend of one of my wheelchair transport drivers was going to tear out the door frames, shore up the fence, build a ramp on my back patio and put in assistive handles and other helpful things to make the place more accessible. We did that after his day job and as he had time, so that meant I had to go there pretty often for short periods of time. I kept getting the same wheelchair transport drivers, at least on the way to my new place or the way back during this time. Larry was one, Wil was another. I had gotten to know many of the wheelchair transport drivers since the negative incident early on, and I never had another situation like that one with any other driver.

I spent the first night in my new place by myself, although I didn't sleep much. I had already scoped out a good half a mile around my place on my trips there, so I knew where the Laundromat, convenient mart, library and a couple of restaurants were near me. I looked forward to exploring more with my dogs on our daily walks around the neighborhood once they would arrive the next day.

When Dan brought them, they barreled through the duplex like couple of horses who had just been let out of the gate for a race. I let them right out the back door and into their new yard. They sniffed every square inch of it. Then they bounded inside and stuck their noses in every nook and cranny of our new living space, taking breaks to run to me with the biggest smiles I had ever seen on their beautiful faces.

I had dreamed of that day for so long, it was hard to believe it was real. They had been my sole motivation to keep going forward since the day nearly 10 months ago that I moved into the homeless project. They had never been far from my heart through so many sleepless, painful nights. They were always what I saw in the glimmers of light that accompanied so many of my episodes of darkness. I was beaming inside and out as I watched them explore our humble abode.

Finally, we were home.

21

Since I was moving to the city of Dunedin, Wil kept insisting that I meet his friend Marilyn who lived near my new place. He just knew that she and I would become friends because of how we feel about our dogs. He was so insistent that it was a little bit uncomfortable. Once my landline phone was turned on, I let him give Marilyn my number and he had given me hers, but I never really intended to call her. To be honest, I was not sure how to interact with new people from a wheelchair—unless they were clients. I seemed to always want to share who I used to be, and it had been so long since I had been that person, I didn't know what to say anymore. I did not want to spend the rest of my wheelchair bound life telling people who I used to be. I did not mind sharing some of that story, but would have liked to have some idea of who I had evolved into to balance it out. Who wants to hear someone go on and on about who they were? I was even getting tired of hearing myself think it. All of this had happened so fast, that I still had not really caught my breath. Maybe I would start breathing again now that my boys were home. Then I could figure out who I had become.

Most of my interactions with new people since this started involved other residents at the homeless project and the nursing home. I guess you could count interactions with wheelchair transport drivers too, but the rest of my interactions with the general public were mixed. I had a few positive encounters mixed with some negatives. I wasn't sure if it was something I was putting out there or if this is just how the general population dealt with people in wheelchairs. Some people spoke to me using a louder voice and slower cadence. Some people would insist on doing everything for me whether I could do it myself or not, and others would approach me in a patronizing or pitying way. Of course, there were the few who tried to take advantage of me thrown in as well. No one could understand what this was like for me, and in that sense, I still felt alone. I wasn't sure I even completely understood what this all had been like for me. In retrospect, I was a great victim a fair portion of the time. I was trying to move beyond that victim mentality, but at this point had not yet realized it was my default perspective. I would find my personal power, then have another setback and fall back into my victim role.

My life was the epitome of unfair and often people who had known me before would validate that for me without my prompting. I certainly tried not to act like a victim by doing things like seeking pity or sympathy, even though I still felt victimized most of the time. I would at least want to be acknowledged some days. I appreciated the acknowledgement now and again of all that I had been through to get to this point. I deliberately did not act as if I was that victim with other people. It was my goal to appear motivated to move forward, well-adjusted, and pleasant to others. If I didn't truly feel that, it was okay because, as they say, fake it until you make it. I believe I was successful at this most of the time.

It was hard to imagine that I was as aware and as conscious of my behavior through the process, but at the same time, I was unaware of how much of this was related to my perception being skewed. My feelings and thoughts didn't come close to matching my behavior. I was hoping my feelings and thoughts would catch up with how I acted in front of other people. They eventually did, but it took a lot of practice. There were always many lessons within my experiences, whether I was interested in the opportunities for growth or not.

So when Wil was trying to push the Marilyn connection, I wasn't sure I was even ready to try to make new friends, and if you remember, I wasn't very skilled at this at any point in my life. I was not skilled at making real friends, anyway. I had many friends/acquaintances, and got along with everybody, but there were few with whom I would show much vulnerability. This issue had absolutely nothing to do with the chair or the illness. I had learned lessons in being vulnerable and with the onset of my illness my vulnerability had magnified. I had worked on that fear of being needy or vulnerable, but would I be able to continue letting myself be vulnerable with others if I wasn't forced to do so? I was coming out of three environments that required that I surrender, to some degree, to being vulnerable and needy. I had also just come out of two environments that, by design, did not allow for me to isolate from others. Now that I was no longer forced to interact socially, would I actively seek that out?

    My phone rang a week or so after I moved in, and it was Marilyn. She told me that Wil would not stop insisting that we connect, so she figured the only way to shut him up was to give me a call. I was not very welcoming of this idea on the phone at all, to put it mildly. I was overtly resistant in fact, but then Marilyn made a valid point that I could not dispute. "Sometimes this is how people meet—through mutual friends," she said. I ended up agreeing to meet up with her on the Pinellas Trail where my dogs would also be introduced to her adorable golden retriever Zeke.

    Wil was right, we were both very similar dog moms. Our outing covered about two miles, north on the trail to downtown, a left turn to the Dunedin Marina and back again. I decided that I really liked her, and it was clear my dogs loved her and loved Zeke, whose face just emanates happy.

    I was feeling guarded but much to my surprise and delight, there was little conversation about my power chair or reasons I was in it. I just gave her a brief synopsis because she didn't know how long I had been in the chair or any of my circumstances. This was only important because I could not answer many of her questions about my interests. Most of the conversation was about our dogs and how much they mean to us. It was as if I was talking with someone who knew me before the chair and illness. She made me feel like an intelligent, regular person with thoughts and ideas. She was asking me questions to try to get to know me—not what I did for a living or anything, but just to know who I was as a person. Marilyn did not seem to care about what I could "do" and instead cared about who I was. I liked that. I liked that a lot. I liked that she could see me, even though I really couldn't see me just yet.

The ironic thing was that, as she was asking me questions, I had no real idea what the answers were anymore. I certainly had no idea of who I was anymore. Her questions about what I liked to do, where I liked to go, etc., left me without answers. I knew what they used to be, but was not sure those fit anymore. I had spent the last three years in a whirlwind and hadn't quite gotten to know the person I had become yet. I knew I had developed different interests in those three years. I knew I felt differently about a lot of things, but hadn't really assimilated the new information well enough to share. My perspective about life was certainly different, but I wasn't able to express how different or in what ways it was different.

All the questions that I couldn't really answer then, were ones I would begin to answer in the coming years by doing new and different things. Had it not been for this arranged meeting, I wouldn't have been as aware that these were things I really needed to explore. I may have stumbled upon the importance of this later on, but this did seem to be something pretty important to figure out before getting too far into this next life chapter. This one interaction also helped me begin to focus on what I could do and what I might want to try to do, rather than focusing on what I couldn't and what I used to like to do. This seemed to create quite a shift in my perspective. I was more forward-focused, than past focused from this one exchange.

22

Developing friendships usually involves going places for lunch, breakfast, or something, which was a struggle for me. I had to use the power wheelchair for everything because I could not stand up from a manual chair to get into a car. That meant I had to use wheelchair transport to meet people, or not meet with them at all. At least those were the limited choices as I saw it then. Scheduling wheelchair transport for a lunch with someone was as tricky as scheduling for a doctor's appointment. You cannot be sure when you will be finished and ready to leave to schedule the pick-up time. If you undershot it, wheelchair transport leaves without you and you could wait a long time before another driver could come get you. If you overshot it, you could be waiting for a really long time to go home. For me, at that point, it seemed easier not to try, rather than to coordinate it. Then there was a matter of whether I would even feel like doing something on the day it was scheduled to happen. I never knew from one day to the next. I was not yet at the point where I was willing to go to such great lengths to develop friendships, even though Marilyn did seem like a person worthy of the effort.

The notion of it being so daunting for us to arrange to have lunch together frustrated Marilyn, and she was determined to figure out a way that we could do it without wheelchair transport. She really was not that tolerant of my excuses for not also trying to figure it out. She was on a mission, with or without my participation. We went to a movie via Wil in his wheelchair transport van, and that was okay for starters. She was certain she could figure out a better way, and refused to be limited by whether Wil could take us. What I know now about Marilyn, who is a lawyer who specializes in medical malpractice, is that once she is presented with a challenge, she becomes almost obsessively focused on it until she figures it out. That is pretty much how this played out and I was impressed at how creative she was getting with potential solutions. There were some ideas that we had to try out to see if they would work because I could not quite envision what she was suggesting.

At the time I met her, she was deciding to buy a new car. She settled on a Honda Element – it has a kind of cube design-- and we found out I could do a sliding transfer from my chair, right onto the back seat floor of the car. Actually, it was almost the perfect height to do it with little effort, and we joked about her being the chauffer since I was riding in the floor of the back seat.

At first, I would try to get myself up onto the seat, but that was exhausting and painful. After we realized that, she would just remove the back seat – one of the car's features-- and I could transfer in and sit on the floor. She continued to try to find a way to make the floor more comfortable, but it really was more comfortable than trying to get up into the seat. My manual wheelchair also easily fit into the car.

I no longer had an excuse not to go to lunch with her, but I would have to let her push me in the manual chair from the car to wherever we were going, and be okay with that. She never made a big deal out of any of it, so I just followed her lead and didn't either. It didn't matter how I felt about it. The important thing was that I was getting out to new places with a new friend.

To her, it had merely been a logistical problem that needed a solution. I was the one who made the big deal emotionally about it. I didn't feel worthy of someone taking such great pains at making something work, at least not in the beginning. I was only used to figuring out how to function with the wheelchair, but that didn't mean I wasn't still sensitive about it. I still always felt in the way and that it was a pain in the ass to take me anywhere. I became a lot less sensitive about it once I saw someone behaving so overtly as if it was a non-issue.

I shared with her my first mall experience in the power chair when she suggested we go to a few thrift stores together. I couldn't get through the aisles of the first one we went to because they were too narrow for the wheelchair. My manual chair was far slimmer than the power wheelchair I had taken to the mall a few years before. We kept trying different thrift stores. As she realized I had not really experienced that much of Florida or our area in the year before getting sick, she would insist we go to different places as well.

Early into the friendship, there were things I intuitively realized that you just do not debate or resist with her. If Marilyn decided she wanted to take me somewhere, then she would be taking me there. My resistance was futile, which was good for me. There was no real purpose being served by resisting it anyway. She wasn't being a bully about it, it was just that my resistance didn't really make any sense for these things.

Of course, that did not stop me from trying to resist entirely, especially in the beginning. I was still having trouble letting go of my old ways of relating to others prior to the wheelchair, and some of the other less than healthy habits of relating since the chair. Here was a person I was interested in being friends with that didn't need rescued, saved or counseled. This would be a friendship of relative equals and I had only had a few of those in my life.

While she wanted to be helpful, she was not overly so and was very respectful of any reasonable boundary I set, and always allowed me to do the things myself that I could do. Marilyn seemed to be able to know that without asking, but when she wasn't sure, she asked.

Actually, she asked a lot of questions about whether something would or could work for me, and sometimes we had to try it to know because I had no idea. This was as new to me as it was to her, but I am not sure either of us understood that fully at the time. Time with her was comfortable and I absolutely fell in love with her dog. My favorite question she would ask when I was sharing something with her, and before she would give any feedback, was "What does that mean to you?"

Marilyn would bring Zeke over to play with and visit my dogs while she and I visited. I couldn't get into her house because she had stairs. She would drive my boys to the marina and get into the water with them in a small beach away from the boat docks. Summers were so hot for Duke and Moré because they are black lab mixes, so driving them meant they would be less tired when they got to the water to play. I would take my power wheelchair from my house to meet them. It was a little over a mile and my chair went 5 mph, so they had some time with each other before I would get there. My boys had loved the water the few times we actually went before I got sick, but only if I was in there with them. Marilyn hoped that they would get in the water with her instead. I hoped so too, and was looking forward to watching the boys get to do something they loved to do.

They did get in the water with her and sometimes they would run right out of the water and we would spent time chasing them around the marina docks when they got away. It was a real challenge playing the cat and mouse game with your dogs when you're in a wheelchair. Duke would often look very upset from the back window of Marilyn's car when he would see me wheeling down the sidewalk alone. After we did this a few times, Duke relaxed a little bit and stuck his head out the same window with Zeke and Moré as they drove away.

One day, she and Zeke were at my house and she said, "You do realize that you have no place for anyone to sit who comes over to visit, don't you?" No one really came to visit me and I hadn't been living there very long at that point. My dad would stop by with lunch or to get my laundry, but I am not sure he ever sat down. I had a bed and my power chair and that was about it. The only seats I could transfer to were my elevated potty chair and my shower bench. It just never occurred to me that someone would want to sit down if they came over. I am not sure it ever occurred to me that anyone would be coming over at all, quite honestly.

I hadn't thought much past getting my dogs back and being in my own place. I still wasn't all that sure I was going to be able to make all of that work. I detected a hint of skepticism from my friends about how I was doing living alone with my dogs. I was determined to make it work, with my dogs, in this new place, so I got an old black loveseat from my neighbor who was giving it away.

Amoré stood at the door whining for Marilyn to come back in after she left. He loved her. He stood there for quite a while before finally laying down with his nose up looking at me, then the door, then back at me. He really liked her and he spent the rest of that night lying by the door. Marilyn and I would develop into great friends over the years. She is now the older sister I never had and her mom became my Mama Ruthie. We often joke about our first phone conversation because we both thought Wil was crazy for being so insistent we meet. It turns out he wasn't crazy at all, but knew enough about us both to know that the potential was there for us to become great friends. Marilyn likes to share the part about my resistance to the whole thing, but mostly to reinforce how far I have come since then.

23

    I had been out of the nursing home almost a year when my anguish over whether I had ALS came to a merciful and somewhat anti-climactic end during a routine appointment with my neurologist, Dr. Frank. Almost nonchalantly, he informed me I might want to get involved with the Spastic Paraplegia Foundation, which raises money for research for Primary Lateral Sclerosis (PLS) and Hereditary Spastic Paraplegia (HSP). Although he said he would continue to monitor my progression for some time to indisputably confirm I had PLS or HSP, he was confident his diagnosis would turn out to be the correct one. That was good enough for me, and time mostly confirmed his diagnosis.

    At last, my chart would no longer say "rule out ALS." I would no longer have to feel the grip of fear in my heart that struck each time I saw those words glaring back at me. The fear of my dogs outliving me would no longer be what so often left me breathless and sleepless at night. Now, the unknown was a known, the mystery solved for the most part.

    I was wracked in pain and spasticity that day, so I was ambivalent about the diagnosis, despite having waited so long to hear it. Yes, there was relief that it wasn't ALS, but having a name for it wasn't going to do anything to make my symptoms go away or to help me manage my life. There is no cure for PLS or HSP, so I knew I was in for a lifelong struggle. I would have to cling to a dream that some future treatment or medical breakthrough might make me alright again, even get me up on my feet and walking.

    Even as Dr. Frank so confidently gave me his probable

diagnosis, pain was shooting through my legs and my shoulder muscles had stiffened so badly I could barely lift my arms. Along with my medications, I had been using visualization exercises, meditation and distraction to help manage the pain. I was again having more difficulty bathing and holding the showerhead to wash and rinse my hair. My range of motion was limited to what was right in front of me or right below waist level.

PLS and HSP are rare motor neuron diseases marked by spasticity, slowly progressive weakness in voluntary muscle movement. It belongs to a group of disorders known as motor neuron diseases. It affects the upper motor neurons – called corticospinal neurons – in the arms, legs and face. It occurs when nerve cells in the motor regions of the cerebral cortex – a thin layer of cells covering the brain -- gradually degenerate, causing movement to be slow and difficult.

The disease often affects the legs first, followed by the body, trunk, arms and hands, and finally the muscles that control speech, swallowing and chewing. Its symptoms include weakness, muscle stiffness and spasticity, clumsiness, slowing of movement, and problems with balance and speech. Because it is a rare condition, no two cases are identical, so some of these symptoms may or may not develop.

The symptoms somewhat mirrored what had happened and was still happening to me, except that my progression was much faster than most and I was much younger than the average age of onset. The reason the diagnosis took so long is that PLS it is often mistaken for ALS and that identifying it requires a tedious process of eliminating other diseases.

It had been 3 years since my symptoms began, but that seemed so terribly long ago, just like the life I used to have and the person I used to be seemed so far away. This thing, this illness, had aged me. I could no longer even remember what it felt like to walk, and images of me running only came in flashes in my dreams, which mostly had become nightmares.

At least now the curtain had been closed on the mystery of what was wrong with me. The ordeal of the search for a diagnosis, which started long before my case was turned over to Dr. Frank, will always be with me. It was a hunt that teased me, taunted me, scared the hell out of me, and then sent me home to stew about it until they were ready to have me come back for more. Some of it is a blur, the doctors, the nurses, the gurneys, the fluorescent lights on the ceilings of so many hospital corridors, the stabs of spinal taps, the machines that pulled me into their cocoons to snap pictures of my brain and my spine.

I had been to rheumatologists, neurologists, internal medicine experts and specialists of every kind. When they were done, they had no more of an idea what was happening to my body than I did. Every now and again, one of the doctors would mention a possible disease and each time I grabbed hold of the name and researched it, only to find out it really didn't fit.

I remember my close encounter with a diagnosis of multiple sclerosis (MS). It came during my final week of tests at Tampa General when I was sent to see the chair of the neurology department, whose specialty was MS. The reason I kept having spinal taps was they were all sure I had MS. I was the right age and was having some symptoms that would come, and then go, and others that were coming so rapidly that it just made the most sense. The problem was the spinal taps and MRIs -- the two main diagnostic indicators of MS -- showed I did not appear to have it.

And other tests showed it wasn't one of the movement disorders such as Parkinson's disease and Ataxia, which is more of a disease of the cerebellum that also causes spasticity and similar symptoms. I remember I asked the doctor after that final day if she thought I was crazy. She performed some of her tests again and said that these things cannot be faked, nor did she think I was crazy. She did send me for yet another test, this one for stiff person syndrome, which is characterized by some of my same symptoms of stiffness, spasms and hyper reflexes. The test was negative.

It was after the expertise of teams of doctors who kept me for three week-long stays at Tampa General failed to figure out what I had, that they sent me to Dr. Frank. When I did a cursory search on him and learned he worked at the Muscular Dystrophy

Association's clinic, I wasn't sure what to think. I didn't know much about muscular dystrophy except that Jerry Lewis does a telethon, and I really couldn't get past the image of Jerry's kids. Then I found out it would take about three months to get in to see him, so my frustration, wondering, worrying would have to simmer for a while longer.

It was mid-July, just before I moved into the homeless project, when I finally got to see him. He was worth the wait.

He was not sure exactly what sort of disease process was working in my body, so we began a more intensive process of elimination that the earlier doctors had started. I had nerve conduction tests, called EMGs, more MRIs of my brain and spinal cord, more labs and we attempted to get some genetic testing, but never got that approved through my insurance.

All of the disease states that could kill me or that were somewhat fixable were ruled out by August 2004, except for one. Because of the rapid progression of my symptoms, there was concern that it could be ALS. Each future appointment with him required me to carry a form from the exam room to the checkout desk with a diagnosis written on it that said, "Rule-out ALS."

Those small written words at the bottom of the page may as well have been the size of a billboard—and all neon in color because they jumped off the page to my eyes much the same way. Regardless of the fact that he and I had discussed that it was probably not ALS, seeing it each time on that form horrified me. ALS has different rates of progression but it most often progresses rapidly and is fatal within a few months or a couple years. My rapid progression was disconcerting and I was more scared than I had ever been.

But in Dr. Frank, I had a neurologist who was willing to figure out the puzzle. He was able to watch how the symptoms were manifesting and evaluate them nearly monthly for about a year, then quarterly after that. He continued to see me regardless of insurance changes and his lack of reimbursement that followed. He finally got me started on some medications to help with the stiffness and pain. He is also the one who helped me get the power wheelchair.

It wasn't hard to see why he was so highly regarded in his field. I know he expended untold energy on my case, and along with his dedication and perseverance he blended in a good measure of kindness on his way to being able to present me my diagnosis.

It took me a while but I gradually warmed up to the idea and got in touch with the PLS support groups he had told me about, which also included support for sufferers of a similar disease called hereditary spastic paraparesis. I found out there was only one other PLS case in my county, a woman named Flora, and began to participate in the PLS online forum.

That's where I learned that no two cases of PLS are the same and just how rare the illness is. It was great to meet others, virtually, who had my illness, but I realized how much younger I was than almost all of them. The average age of the onset of PLS is 50 and I was 32 when it first started.

Flora, her husband and I would go out to eat and they would help me to do some things around my place. In the forums, I finally met another younger person. Her progression was similar to mine as well. Our stories actually mirrored each other, so we started to talk outside of the support forums.

Sarah lived in North Carolina and was about my age. For her, speech and swallowing continued to be issues, whereas for me, swallowing at night was an issue. Sarah, Flora and a few others in various places around the world were not ones who wanted to focus on our symptoms or limitations. We wanted to focus on figuring out how to enhance our quality of life regardless of the symptoms. Sometimes the forum got a little too symptom-focused for me. I was curious about what everyone else was doing for their spasticity and what was working. The medications were not appearing to do much except make me dopey.

Now that I knew what I had, I was determined to try anything that might help me better manage my pain and spasticity. I was especially interested in any kind of physical therapy that when combined with my medication might make a difference.

24

I awakened one morning a few months after being back with my boys with what was probably the best idea I had had for a while. I wondered if physical therapy in a pool would help loosen up my shoulders so that I could better use my arms. I had an appointment that day with Dr. Frank for Botox injections in my legs, not the cosmetic Botox but a kind that paralyzes the muscle where it is injected as a treatment for spasticity. It was expensive and impractical to have it done regularly. Anyway, as he was injecting my legs I talked with him about how much difficulty I was having using my arms and how the limited range of motion in my shoulders was creating more movement challenges for me. I mentioned my water therapy idea to him, and to my delight, he said it certainly could help and gladly gave me a referral for it.

At that time, I did not yet have Medicare and had Florida's Medicaid share of cost program, which meant I was pretty limited in terms of what complementary assistance I could get for water therapy sessions. I found out that I could get only six sessions total, and the first of those would be an evaluation, rather than an actual in-the-pool therapy session. I figured anything was better than nothing, and it was worth trying. I then found out that the only pool therapy available in Pinellas County was in St. Petersburg. In terms of wheelchair transport, this was an all day ordeal to schedule a trip there, get to the appointment and then wait for the return transport to arrive to bring me back up to the north part of the county.

I was willing to do it, but worried about how the fatigue from making the trip would affect my ability to do day-to-day things. In addition to that, I would be exerting effort in a pool for physical therapy. As things were since I had gotten out of the nursing home, it was taking me all day to get a very short list of tasks accomplished. I decided to spread out the sessions over a few weeks to allow time to recuperate between them and still be able to bathe, cook and clean.

I don't remember the evaluation session, but do remember liking a therapist named Lori and hoping she knew what she was doing. I was concerned there was no lift to get me from the chair to the water, but was assured that they would get me in there. Lori would have a student with her, and both she and her student were interested in learning more about my illness. Since it is rare and each case seems to be different in its presentation, they were unfamiliar with it.

My first pool session would have been comical if it wasn't so discouraging. I wondered if it was going to be worth all of the effort and energy. They put a floatation belt around my waist that was supposed to keep me somewhat stable in the water—I think that was assuming several other things that I was unable to do. I had been in a chair at that point for nearly three years and since almost the entire year of symptoms and illness progression involved no treatment at all, I was not in great shape. My left leg had hardly any muscle mass left. I was underweight and just about all my major muscles were atrophied. My feet had contorted from all of the spasticity in my legs, so they didn't stand flat anymore unless there was no weight or pressure on them. I had not been able to stand at all for close to 18 months.

One of the young strong physical therapists had to lift me out of my chair and carry me down the two steps into the water where I was supposed to hold onto the side to try to stand. I kept falling over. Because I was in the water with the flotation belt, I felt like a weeble-wobble. I had no control over where I went at all. I felt like I had no control over what my body would do, even if I was holding on to the side. Lori and her student kept helping me get back upright. I couldn't quite keep my feet under me because they were twisted to the sides. I could only put weight on the back, outer side of my right heel and really no weight on any part of the left foot.

Noticing this, Lori commented, so I told her about my feet and how long they had been that way and how I felt certain if I could get my calf muscles to relax enough, that the tiny muscles all in my feet might also relax. At any rate, I wasn't sure I could walk in the pool unless my feet could somehow be fixed. My primary goal was not to walk in the pool, however, but to be submerged enough that my shoulders could benefit from the water's healing powers. When submerged in water, the muscles are far less contracted than they are out of the water because of the effects of gravity.

Lori got an idea as I was talking and suddenly she was telling her student and me what she was thinking. We got my feet turned the right way and they proceeded to stand on them under the water. Lori was on one foot and the student was on the other one. I am not sure I remember how long they did this, but as I recall, we did little else that session. It was a bit painful, but I am sure it would have hurt far more if we had been doing it on dry land. The water made my arms feel better, and I was even hopeful that their plan to fix my feet would work.

What happened in my third session totally changed my perspective of my illness, my prognosis and turned out to be another one of those special times that changed the course of my life.

I still needed lifted into the pool by the young strong physical therapist and Lori and her student again stood on my feet for a bit once I got in, even though they were already much better than they were. We did some exercises, although I don't recall what they were. The next thing I knew I was standing up, and I mean standing upright on my feet. I was holding onto Lori, the student or the side of the pool, but I was standing just the same.

Somewhere in the course of conversation and exercises, the

topic of atrophied muscles came up. I only remember asking Lori, "Is it even possible to reverse atrophy?" I remember her response even more, "Well...yes, it is possible, but..." I think she said something about it taking a lot of work and a lot of time, and probably more about muscle death because of disease processes, but I honed in on the "yes" and from that point forward knew what my new mission was going to be. I had been told that I would not likely walk again. Up to that point, I believed that the damage that had been done could not be undone, so my mind was completely blown when I realized that perhaps I could reverse the course of my atrophied muscles. If I could do that, then I would get stronger, and if I kept doing the pool who knows what I could accomplish.

I was thrilled about standing in the pool. I talked about it non-stop all the way home with my driver, and when I got home, I told my dogs all about it and how I couldn't wait to see what happened next.

My fourth session was even more incredible. My feet didn't require anyone to stand on them and I was able to venture away from Lori, the student and the sides of the pool and actually walk a few steps in the water. I could not believe it. I did not want to get out of the pool ever, ever, ever again. At that point, I was talking to Lori about pools in my part of the county, and what I could continue to do on my own after our sessions were over.

I walked in the water. I really walked in the water. I called and emailed just about everyone I knew. I asked my dad if he thought there was a way to have a house designed that was filled with water up to my waist? He shared my excitement, but I think he thought I had lost it a little bit.

For my fifth session, I brought a little video camera that my brother had given me for Christmas. I was feeling pretty confident and had the young, strong physical therapist come in, but not to carry me into the pool---to watch me try to walk into the pool. I had it in my mind that I wanted to try to do those two steps that led into the water. That's right, I did. The girl who was told to get used to being in a wheelchair the rest of her life was walking her happy ass into the physical therapy pool.

Okay, so it wasn't all that. I pretty much used my arms on the railing and the physical therapist for balance to get myself down those two steps into the pool. But it was close enough to walking into the pool for me. After I got in, I continued to walk in the water with much more stability than the previous session. I was very weak, however, so I made a mental note to not get too carried away. I had Lori video tape it for me so I could show Dr. Frank. I wanted to figure out how to email it to everyone, so I could show it to the world. My final session did involve me walking from my chair into the pool without anybody helping me. I still used the rail like it was a lifeline, but I did it by myself just the same.

When I worked as a homeless outreach therapist, I had written several letters for clients to get scholarship memberships to the YMCA. It allowed them to join the YMCA and use the facilities at a reduced fee. Between my fifth and sixth sessions, I checked into the application process and whether they had a lift into the pool. While I could take two small steps into the pool at the small physical therapy pool, a real pool would take considerably more strength, coordination and balance, and I didn't have it—at least not yet.

I ended up getting the scholarship membership to the YMCA in Clearwater and proceeded to go at least once a week through the summer and fall. I would take wheelchair transport there in the mornings. The lifeguard used the lift to get me into the pool. The lift put me into the deep end, so I was diligent in wearing the floatation belt Marilyn had lent me.

I had no idea if I could actually swim, but felt certain drowning was not an option. I would work my way from the deep end to the shallow end, which proved to be no easy feat on those first few trips. I had never been a strong swimmer and was lacking confidence in my strength. I was often there during a water aerobics class, so I would have to get over to the opposite side of the Olympic sized pool into the lanes reserved for swimmers doing laps.

At first, I thought I might have to make sure I was there at a time when there was no aerobics class because the waves they generated were considerable. These were not small women doing the water aerobics class, and they generally had a pretty large group. As I was walking back and forth in the shallow end of the lane, I was using the wall to help me because of the women exercising really stirred up the water. I wanted to walk and walk and walk without any waves, but I did not often get to do that. But by the third or fourth time, I realized that their waves were actually helping me develop better balance and coordination. The added water resistance from the waves was also helping me develop muscle strength.

After the fifth or sixth time, I found myself wondering if someday I could participate in their aerobics class rather than walking. I enjoyed walking so much that I often had to give myself special rules to make sure I got out of the water before I hurt myself from doing too much. Imagine going from not considering being able to walk again to being able to stand, and then walk in the water. Then imagine entertaining the notion of doing water aerobics. I could hardly wrap my head around the shift in my way of thinking about my world.

To get to the pool, I had to wheel past the gym where all the workout equipment was. Each time I went by I allowed myself to imagine one day being back on an exercise bike, elliptical machine or treadmill. Wouldn't that be cool, I would say to myself. I also had to wheel the racquetball courts, and the smells coming from them brought back memories of playing racquetball every week with my friend Patty when I taught a night class at Marshall University. I wondered if they had wheelchair racquetball and how that would work. Sometimes I would see flyers on the walls for wheelchair basketball. I had a ways to go to make my arms strong enough to take a shot, but I entertained the thought just the same.

My arms were doing consistently better with the water's help. I was feeling like my legs were getting stronger too. They were still spastic when I tried to move them too much and sometimes they would just jump around. While I wasn't deluded into thinking that my illness wouldn't continue to progress, I did believe that I could improve the quality of my life now that I had the pool in my life.

Even though I was walking in the water, I no longer had the memory of what it felt like to walk. I didn't remember how it felt to have the smooth movement from my waist, hips, quads, hamstrings, calves, ankles and down to my feet. I couldn't conjure what that felt like anymore. I would watch breakfast at Wimbledon and watch them run around the court trying to remember what that felt like. I would watch golf on television and found myself fixating on how they walked around the course, and try with all my might to remember what that would feel like. If the brained processed what we imagined as if it was happening, then I needed to be able to imagine being able to walk on land. I was frustrated that I couldn't remember how it felt.

By late fall, the pool was too chilly for me. The drawback to this YMCA was that the pool isn't heated and it is covered, so the sun cannot really help heat it either. I tried going from the pool to the hot tub because I would shiver with cold soon as I got out of the pool and my whole body would be in spasm. I decided the benefits of building muscle mass was still worth it for as long as it was warm enough. I continued going into the early winter months but not as frequently.

In those later days of going to the YMCA pool, I wasn't using the lift anymore to get in the water. I also wasn't using the floatation belt. I could go from the chair, to the ladder and ease my way down the ladder and actually sort of swim to the shallower end of the pool. I sometimes needed the lift to get out of the pool, but that even got fewer and farther in between. One day, I even ventured into the workout room. It was tight in there with the wheelchair, but now that I could do a standing transfer, I wondered if I could ride the stationary bicycle. It felt awkward to get on the bike from the chair, particularly with the entire room watching me do it. I couldn't seem to get the bike programmed correctly, so I just tried a few rotations of the pedals. I wasn't quite ready for the bike. My feet wouldn't stay on the pedals at all and I felt like I would just fall off the seat.

I continued to work at home to build my strength in hopes

of being able to stand and walk out of the water. By July, I had my walker parked by my kitchen counter and I would spent time standing there with the walker behind me and the counter in front of me. I did this every single day and sometimes several times a day until I could also do something else while I was standing there. Eventually, I could stand and cook something that didn't take long and could do a few dishes. By the end of August, I was really wondering if I could take some steps safely. Since I lived alone with my dogs, I didn't want to fall and end up in worse shape than I started in.

    My one dog Duke had helped me up in the early months of my illness without any training and he had been watching me closely during my standing adventures in the kitchen all summer. I figured he would help me if I fell and that I would try it in the living room where there was more space, fewer things to hit my head on and carpet for a softer fall. I had no intention of falling, however.

    I called for Duke, he came and I had the walker ready in front of my wheelchair. I stood up, got my bearings while making eye contact with Duke. I took about four or five steps forward with the walker and then back to the chair. My living room isn't that big. I did it. I didn't fall. I took steps on land. I used my legs more than my arms like I am pretty sure it should be with a walker. Okay, so my walk was more like a hobble but I did it just the same and had a feeling that my life was soon going to change a lot.

25

When I started pool therapy sessions in 2006, Marilyn, Karen and Dan got to be the first to hear about my feet being flattened and then about me "walking" in the water. Walking in the water translated later to me being able to go more places and do more things with people because I was able to transfer more safely. I had been to Marilyn's house in my power chair, but could only go through the garage door and out its back door, to hang out on the patio below her raised wooden deck. I would walk the boys over and she would make breakfast or coffee, and make us a little seating area on that little patio space. There were stairs at each entrance of her house. The back and garage entrance had only two steps up to the deck, which would be the easiest way to try to get inside.

After I had been practicing standing and felt strong enough, I went to her house to see if I could get closer to inside. I had been a bit nervous testing my new hobbles at home alone, so trying it with people made good sense. I didn't actually share my intention with Marilyn to hear her tell this story. She invited me over one evening to meet a friend of hers who was in town. I took my power chair over to her house and went in through the garage, just as I had always done. Marilyn swears I said nothing to them outside of hello and casual conversation before I got up to hobble over to where they were sitting on the other side of her pretty large deck.

When I stood up to try to take those steps up to the deck

using the railing, I was looking around at how different it all looked from a standing position. I made it up the two steps and that is when Marilyn saw me and realized that I wasn't sitting in the chair. She was getting ready to move things over to my side of the deck with her back turned while I climbed the stairs, and that is how she missed me doing it. I had shared with her on the phone that I was hobbling around the house a little more, but she hadn't actually seen it for herself yet.

    Now I was on the deck, but I stood there frozen. I was afraid to let go of the railing because where they were standing seemed so far away from where I was. It may as well have been an open football field, even though it was really only about 15 feet. There was nothing for me to hold onto along the way, and perhaps if I had thought this all the way through, I might have realized such a flaw in my unspoken plan. I really just wanted to see if I could get up those two steps and hadn't considered what I would do next if I could.

    Once Marilyn saw me, she first went into helpful mode almost automatically, but then she realized that I was standing in front of her. She arranged chairs for me to hold onto so that I could go farther because that was the only thing we could think of to do next. She was spotting me as I hobbled closer to where she and her friend were on the deck. I hobbled from chair to chair. My walking was stiff and Frankenstein-ish, so I refer to it as hobbling rather than truly walking.

    She was getting emotional and I was marveling at how different her deck looked, how different everything looked, from a standing position. I still wasn't saying anything aloud, perhaps because I was also having to concentrate to make sure that my feet were coming far enough off of the deck each step of the way. I had known Marilyn for over a year at this point and never gave a second thought about whether she was tall or short. Everyone is tall when you are sitting down. Marilyn gave me a hug and I just blurted out, "I didn't realize you were so short." It was obvious that I was not the only one who was surprised to have said that, and I couldn't tell if she was offended or not.

    She laughed a little, but was still emotional about me being upright. I immediately started trying to explain myself. She really was not short, just about an inch shorter than I was. But, boy did I feel about six feet tall compared to how I felt from a seated position in the wheelchair. Everyone was tall and that is just how it had been. When I talked with someone from my chair my view was usually limited to their stomach, or worse, their crotch if they were tall.

    Marilyn has brought up that story many times since then. Neither of us can remember what happened next, but I would venture to guess that sangria was involved. They both walked me part of the way home since I was in the chair with no lights and I stayed a lot longer than I had planned. It had started raining, so Marilyn put a poncho over me that also covered the back of my chair. I could now get into Marilyn's house and just needed to bring a walker with me the next time I went.

    The pool therapy and my continued efforts at going to the YMCA to walk in the water had helped my arms a lot. Now I could actually start to do some restorative physical therapy exercises with them to try to develop some strength and work on reversing atrophied muscles. The physical therapy assistant from the nursing home had sent me home with some resistance bands, and I used those some each day, but that was pretty boring when I could be doing something more fun or practical. I had already turned my daily chores into physical therapy activities and it seemed to be working pretty well for me.

    I woke up one morning and decided to take my basketball up to the elementary school to try to shoot baskets at the kiddie rim from the wheelchair or maybe even standing in front of the wheelchair. I took the boys with me, tied them up on another basketball post and proceeded to wheel up close to the backboard to toss the ball up there. At first, the ball wasn't hitting anything—not the net, and certainly not the backboard or rim. I wasn't sure this was going to work because I was spending more time chasing after the ball than anything resembling physical therapy. I kept at it and the second time we went, I was able to hit the bottom edge of the backboard, so I did that for a few repetitions on each side with each arm as if I was doing a layup. The next time, I was getting the ball a bit higher and by the fourth trip, I was getting the ball high enough on the backboard to bank it into the rim at least once. I was really shooting baskets. I had missed shooting baskets a lot. My arms were getting stronger too.

    Not much longer after that, I was able to use my walker at Marilyn's house to hobble around. My dogs loved her backyard, and as I got more and more stable, we would spend a great deal more time there. Of course, this new hobbling meant that I needed even more furniture in my place. The first thing I realized was that I needed a desk chair. I was no longer wheeling around in the duplex doing everything from the wheelchair and it never occurred to me that to sit in front of my computer, I would need something to actually sit on. My neighbor worked as a maintenance man at a nursing home, which would often throw things and replace them something new. I mentioned that I could really use an office chair, so he brought me one. It was made for a very overweight person, but it worked just fine and was better than nothing. I could never have imagined, even six months earlier, that I would be in need of furniture for myself. I never imagined I would ever be walking again, even though I kept dreaming about it.

    I would dream that I was walking around. The dream would be flowing along nicely until I realized that I was walking. At that point in my dream, I would panic and begin to do my wounded soldier crawl to find my wheelchair. I had a couple dreams about losing my wheelchair while I was living at the homeless project, but it was a dream I was having repeatedly since I was back with my dogs. I found waking up from the panic of losing the chair bothersome at night since deep sleep was hard to come by. In the dream, I couldn't actually see the motion of walking, nor did I feel it. My legs often weren't even visible in the dreams, so I was more or less floating around as a standing person. In my waking life, I couldn't remember what it felt like to walk, so I gathered that was probably the reason for it.

    By the summer of 2005, back with my dogs in my new place, those dreams came almost every other night and I would be left exhausted. I spent a great deal of energy during the day reminding myself that walking was not supposed to happen again. At the time, I interpreted the dreams to be my inability to let go of the idea of being an ambulatory person. I had decided they were more prevalent because I was in a new environment and afraid of waking up and trying to get out of bed the way I used to be able to—by standing up. Since then, I have been caught saying, "I never dreamed I would be walking again," which isn't necessarily true since I had dreamed I would walk again and dreamed it often both at the homeless project and at the nursing home.

But I knew I wasn't dreaming when I was standing at a podium in the fall of 2006 as the coordinating speaker at retreat for women who suffered from either what I had or the similar disorder called hereditary spastic paraparesis (HSP).

The retreat came about in conversations with online support groups for people with both diseases. It would be a retreat to deal specifically with women's issues common to both chronic illnesses. I agreed to help plan it with a woman who had HSP. I had done quite a few women's psycho-educational groups back in my working days, and was looking forward to tailoring the sessions and speakers to our illnesses and issues. I solicited my former therapist Jenny – the one I couldn't wait to show my light-in-the-dark painting – to give a talk on assertiveness. Having her there provided a special moment for me, which came when I was able to hug her standing up.

We named the retreat "New Moves: an empowerment retreat for mobility challenged women." We did the retreat in Tampa during in mid-October. Flora, the PLS sufferer I met along with her husband on my first foray into the online forum, helped me copy and put together packets for the retreat that included information I had gathered for my two talks, and outlines for each speaker's presentations. The planning and preparation was exhausting and frustrating. I remember complaining a lot and wondering why I had taken on so much responsibility. But I knew why I did it. This type of retreat was right up my alley and I wanted to make sure we included what I found to be important to women with mobility issues. The program dealt thoroughly with all the issues I had struggled with and was still struggling with as I muddled through my life. I was also thankful that it became a team effort because there is no way I could have done all that I did without the rest of the team.

One of the sessions I led was on self-image, the other on coping with loss. As you have noticed so far, my self-image took a beating when I was in the wheelchair and it wasn't at all great before the chair. I presumed that might be the case with other women with chronic, progressive illnesses and it certainly was a topic of interest for all those who were there.

In my loss group, I talked about how cyclical the grieving process was each time the symptoms progressed. Each new symptom, or worsening of an existing symptom, was accompanied by a functional impairment. We often had to give up something in our life as it occurred. For me, it was a rapid process. I was actually trying to adjust in the opposite direction now with my new found abilities to stand and walk, or more accurately hobble. I allowed time at the end of my talk for participants to anonymously write down losses they were struggling with and we went through them as a group.

Both groups provided opportunities to become more aware of what each woman was struggling with in these areas and at the end and in the packet, strategies were provided to help with each area. We wanted everyone to leave with more tools than they came in with and to feel empowered by the experience.

I loved being back in front of a group of people talking about something that was important and helpful. I loved even more that I could do it standing up. The standing part became a bit of a challenge after the first session because my ankles were really hurting. It hadn't been that long since I first began hobbling after all my work in the pool, so my legs were not used to it. I was also having some brain issues because I was still on 14 different medications, most of them sedating. I realized I wasn't stable enough standing to try to write on the flip chart very well, or maybe the flip chart stand was not stable enough for me to lean on.

I wasn't sure if what I said up there made sense, but was told afterwards that it did. Once I get on a roll talking about something in front of an audience, I don't always remember exactly what I said or how I said it. That is how it always was in my classes too.

The event succeeded in moving all of us beyond our symptoms to imagine what was possible as we learned to better manage our illnesses.

It was empowering for me for several reasons. I hadn't been able to focus that well, so planning it helped me to learn to do that again. It made me feel useful in both planning it and being the presenter for the topics we selected; it gave me a purpose beyond caring for myself and my dogs, which was all I had done for a few years. It was the longest I had stood up and hobbled around, and while it was exhausting and painful, it was so awesome; and I was able to share my knowledge, experience and expertise with a group of women who were struggling just like me.

I had come so far from the darkness that engulfed me at the homeless project and the fiasco that was the nursing home. I was finding places again in my heart for hope, but never could I have imagined the wondrous thing that awaited me.

26

About two months after our retreat, right around my 36th birthday, my two-year wait for Medicare was over, and I was able to begin my search for a doctor to implant in me a pump that would feed the drug baclofen directly into my spinal fluid. In the simplest terms, what I have makes my muscles contract as if I were in a constant state of flexion. If you have ever flexed a bicep and held it like that for as long as you could, you may have experienced a feeling all of the muscles tightening. For me, that flexion doesn't release, creating spasticity, an unrelenting symptom of my disease. The drug baclofen helps relax and de-contract my muscles.

I had been taking baclofen all along orally but it was often ineffective and contributed to making my feel sleepy. The dramatic exception to that came when I had it injected into my spinal canal during the brief intrathecal pump trial during my second month at the nursing home. Though the trial lasted only four hours, it was a beautiful four hours, marked by a significant improvement in my spasticity. I had no way of knowing then what it could mean, but I tucked the memory away as if I were locking a diamond necklace in a bank vault for safe keeping.

It was now time to be rewarded for my patience during the 18-months I waited for the Medicare I needed to get it. The pump representative who oversaw my trial had said at the time I would be an excellent candidate to have one put in. In all of my research on intrathecal baclofen pumps and in all of the anecdotal information I had received from other people with the pumps, the most important part was selecting the right doctor. The doctor needed to have plenty of experience implanting them or there could be complications.

Finding a doctor did not prove to be an easy task, especially one who would accept what Medicare would reimburse. I had read just about everything I could about how to select a doctor because apparently some doctors are willing to do it even without having much experience doing it. I didn't want to have the complications I was hearing about from others. This surgery is considered minor, but there is a catheter from the pump to the spinal canal to deliver the baclofen. If any part of the subcutaneous placement of the pump or the catheter placement isn't done correctly, any number of problem scenarios could result.

I found the only pain management group in my area, but they weren't on my insurance plan as in-network. The billing specialist was great and decided to try to work with the private insurance group I had to manage my Medicare to make me in-network since there wasn't another option within an hour's drive for me. Once that was squared away, I had the appointment to discuss getting an implant.

At the first appointment, they showed me all my pump options. I had only read about Medtronic brand pumps and had never heard about the Codman brand, which is made by Johnson and Johnson. I wasn't thrilled about the battery situation with Medtronic brand because that meant a surgery would have to done every four years to change the battery. The Codman pump didn't run on batteries. It ran on a gas that was inside the cylinder of the pump and this gas operated on body temperature. It was not necessary to have additional surgery and it came with a lifetime warranty. I chose the Codman. The Codman selection had a different trial process, and one that required a few days stay in the hospital.

During the stay, a temporary catheter tip would be surgically placed in the intrathecal space of the spinal column. Each day, the doctor would come in and increase the dose and we would monitor the results.

I was 36 years old and relatively healthy, so I focused little on the possible adverse events that could occur with the trial. I had read about issues others had with the pumps in the PLS and HSP forums, but I wasn't concerned. This was going to help me to get off some of the sedating medication and get my functioning brain back eventually. Since I could hobble around already, I wondered just how much more I would be able to do with the pump once I had it. I hadn't expected to be able to do much more than I already was doing, but to be able to do it more comfortably. First things first, though, the Codman pump trial.

The following is what I wrote in my blog on the third day of my four-day trial:

The Perfect Day:

It was Wednesday, February 14, 2007, and I awoke in the hospital having had an actual night's sleep! Having signed my life away, I was able to leave the floor to go to the "leper colony" or the smoking area, but was unable to secure a cup of coffee before I left. Still a bit on the sleepy side, and it still being a bit on the dark side out, I wandered into the smoking area in my power chair seeing no one. Oops, there was an older man sitting in the back far corner and I had to squint to see him after I heard "happy valentine's day, lady." Remembering it was actually Valentine's Day, I returned the sentiment and thanked him for being so nice so early in the morning. He left and others came, all of whom were wished a happy valentine's day from me now upon their entrance. A nice woman on her way to work in the ER even gave me her coffee. Smiles were everywhere regardless of circumstances once they heard those magic words, "Happy Valentine's Day!"

My day was already going well as I headed back up to my floor, wishing all I saw a happy valentine's day along the way. The nurse's shifts had changed on my floor, so a completely new group of folks got to hear it from me.

My doc came in to increase the dosage again on my pretend intrathecal baclofen pump and I was excited to see what this increase would bring. The dose the day before had me walking the hallways a bit farther from the walls than the day before. Today, there was a definite improvement in balance and walking. Still wishing Valentine's to all who hadn't heard it (and some over again as I had lost track of who was who by mid-morning), I began to have this strange, but nearly reminiscent sensation going from my feet back up my legs. I walked around some trying to figure it out and determined finally that I was using my whole feet to walk. Now, I know that sounds strange and I had to explain it so that I was not transferred to the psych ward because I was smiling like a small child at Christmas. I have not been able to use the muscles in my feet to walk for 4 years. My latest walking has been on my heels only because of the muscle rigidity in my legs and feet, which is why I called it hobbling.

Now I am thrilled with this new dose and it has only been a few hours! I was continuing to share valentine's wishes, but now with an even larger grin than I had before...

The smiles on my face had contorted to a serious, puzzled look as I struggled to identify the new sensations as I walked down the halls. Let me interject here to add that it is unusual for people in the telemetry/neurological unit to be walking up and down the hallways, so I got more than my share of "may I help you" questions. I simply replied, "no thank you, I am just practicing re-learning how to walk." That would be that, and I do not think anyone really wanted to ask me more about that. It did seem that having a patient in the hallway was not their ideal situation.

Because I only wanted to keep walking around, I had to slow myself down and be off my legs for at least an hour in between my walks up and down the halls. My legs are still not as strong and the muscles that were being loosened certainly have not been used for a while.

Back to my perfect day...my balance continued to improve, but I was having difficulty getting used to my new feet and had to take great care in not tripping as I was walking. I was walking without walls by noon, but quite slowly and deliberately. Thinking about each step I took, I was trying to figure out how in the hell I had been hobbling around without the use of my whole feet before this procedure. As the hours passed, I was thinking less and walking with larger steps and going faster than before. I purposefully would walk smack in the center of the hall so I had no walls to bounce off, nor did I need the walls anymore. The nurses on the day shift were great and as needed, they just ran around me to get where they needed to go...the doctors on the floor were not quite as forgiving and I had to cede to their path. This was good because I needed to see if I could change direction as easily as I was walking. Um, not quite so sturdy initially, but after a while and around four o'clock in the afternoon, I was actually quite good at moving out of the way of oncoming.

The day was passing quickly. I knew that this dose was the dose. I savored each and every second and by the second half of the day, it actually felt like a completely different day. I nearly had to pinch myself because it was so surreal. Around 5:30pm, I took a stroll down the hallway. There was this odd sensation occurring around my hips and top of my butt and I really could not figure out what it was. I continued my second lap around the floor when suddenly I realized that my hips were swaying in natural movement with my feet and legs. I kept walking because I thought I might be imagining it or that it might stop.

I was not imagining it; I had my natural sway back. I, at that point of realization, remembered again, what it felt like to walk normally. Having not walked for nearly four years, I had lost that memory and could not even conjure it when watching others walk. I now knew what it felt like! I really could not believe it and told anyone who would listen. If I had to design how this day would go, I would have sorely fallen short of the amazing feats of the day. (No pun intended)

My legs were surely tired after all the walking of the day, so I decided to rest them and then became lost in thoughtful reflection of this day. I never dreamed this trial dose would be so amazing. I never imagined that one day, from beginning to end, could be THIS wonderful to experience. Although it continued to feel like it was happening to someone else, I also knew the reality of the trial being over in the morning. I thought little of that, but could not help but be filled with awe and then fear that my life as I have known and adjusted to it, would be changing dramatically with the surgical implant of this pump. So many things to think about, but all I could really think about was this day and how magical it was for me. I sought out others who had shared this wonderful day with me...my nurse, the ER nurse, the SW who had been dodging me in the hallways. Nearly tearful, I thanked them for participating in my perfect day. They were nearly tearful and thanked me for reminding them of the many things they take for granted. A final Valentine's wish went to them all.

The following morning, Thursday, would be final day of the trial. The dose actually bottomed out my blood pressure and I nearly passed out, so it was removed and I was heading back home. An hour or so after the pretend pump catheter was removed, I was actually doing worse than I had been doing before the trial began. This was called rebound spasticity and it would take 12-36 hours for me to return to my normal level of spasticity.

Even though I understood why, it was a little freaky to experience. All I could think was what if it doesn't return to my normal? Furthermore, after such great gains the day before, I am not sure I remembered what my normal was before we started the trial.

After the trial, you have to wait about a month to get the pump implanted. The back area needs time to heal. **Before we could schedule the implant, I had to have a psychological evaluation completed.** I found that strange, but apparently there are people who will have unnecessary surgery. I had never come across any clients like that, but tried to hurry to get this evaluation done just the same. The psychologist enjoyed hearing my story and gave his blessing for the implanted pump. Then the surgery was scheduled.

The month of waiting went pretty quickly because I had to get caught up on cleaning and organizing before the surgery. This surgery was minimally invasive, but the back area would likely be sore and would make it a challenge to get the normal daily things done. My head was spinning with the possibilities of my life after the pump implant. I will admit that I was concerned about a few things, but not any of the things you might expect.

I had learned to slow down in my life after having struggled for years to do so. I was more present and more grateful for everything, particularly the little things. I was afraid I would lose these lessons, particularly about the value of stillness, if my life were going to change as dramatically as the perfect day had indicated it would. How would I manage adapting again to a different way of being? When I wasn't wondering these things, I was dreaming about actually walking my dogs on foot rather than from the power chair.

The first scheduled pump implant didn't happen. We were all there at the hospital but the pump representative was a no show. There had been a miscommunication with the doctor's office and the pump representative's office. It was just as well because I was a nervous wreck. My head was spinning so fast with everything I had been thinking about that I really wasn't in a good head space for the surgery.

It was rescheduled for the following week, so I had seven days to get myself calmed down and better prepared for it. I would deal with whatever happens next as it happened and not a moment before. Once I got back to thinking that way, I was ready.

I had them take out a significant amount of spinal fluid to send to a research program in Massachusetts when they implanted my pump. The research project was the development of a PLS registry and it was an opportunity to have them take the spinal fluid while I was having a surgery anyway, but it did make the first few days after surgery a bit worse for me.

The surgery left me with severe headaches, and troubling pain in my back and torso. In the days immediately after getting the pump, I wasn't able to do much more than the hobbling I was doing before. I knew that figuring out the pump dose would not be that simple, and each month the pump had to be refilled, so we could adjust the dose upward at precise rate. It seemed to take me quite a while to heal, although I wasn't sure what normal really was for healing from this type of surgery.

As the months passed I was able to get around better until

finally my feet and hips were all moving in sync. I used a walker for long walks, and a cane if I wasn't going far. I still walked the dogs in the power chair because I wasn't stable enough on my feet yet to handle the sudden direction changes and yanks that go with dog walking.

By late summer, I only used a cane and it might have been for security more than necessity.

27

The mountain bike in Marilyn's garage was calling to me. It was late summer and I was house sitting, and Zeke sitting while she and her boyfriend were traveling through Vietnam. It was like one I used to have, and I was wondering if I could ride it. The adventurer in me that had been dormant so long was stirring again.

When I mentioned my bike riding notion to Marilyn when she called to check in from her travels, she said "Tawny, if you can ride that mountain bike, then you can have it...but please be careful." Her offer was all the incentive I would need. I would set out the next morning.

My riding partner would be a 13-year-old girl that Marilyn had solicited to help me walk the dogs. We put our helmets on and started out on the Pinellas Trail, a 20-foot-wide strip of asphalt that covers close to 50 miles. We headed north through downtown Dunedin toward the Dunedin Causeway intersection about three miles away. We got there and my young friend had already asked me a dozen times if I was sure I was okay to continue. I wasn't that comfortable, but was so excited about actually riding a bike again that I wasn't about to stop.

It was the look on my face that was prompting her concern. My face didn't look like the face of someone having a good time. It was the strained, uncomfortable face I always get when I am concentrating. I managed to relax a bit as we continued the next quarter mile to the base of an elevated pedestrian bridge that spans the main road. The bridge allows the trail to continue on the other side of the main road so that the walkers, runners and bikers do not have to cross traffic. Getting to the main span of the bridge required going up a steep incline. My legs did pretty well in a low gear, but I ended up walking the bike most of the way. My chaperone was great, waited for me half way up and walked next to me.

The next feat I faced was going down the other side. I was still a little bit uncomfortable, but loved the idea of going down a hill full speed. I was flying. I didn't slow down until the bike's momentum slowed on its own near a produce stand where my friend stopped for a soda. It had been exhilarating, the speed was amazing and I wanted to do it again and again, like a kid on his first big slide.

My legs felt weak and a bit wobbly while I was standing off the bike at the produce stand, so I told my friend it was probably best to head back home. So, back we went up the bridge and zoomed down the other side. I secretly hoped the momentum of going down would get me all the way home because I was tuckered out.

We went a bit slower on the way back. I was definitely more comfortable and relaxed, or maybe I was just too tired to be tensed up. We logged more than eight miles that day and I really didn't have any problems at all. I couldn't wait to tell Marilyn how I earned her bike honestly and had a witness to back me up.

I got to tell her all about it the next day during one of her check-in calls. The first thing she said was how happy she was for me, but also said she had a hard time comprehending that I could ride a bike that far, or ride a bike at all for that matter. I assured her that I really did it but she said she would have to see it for herself when she got back.

I brought my own bike when I moved to Florida but riding it was something I had put off doing until it was no longer an option when my symptoms began. I ended up giving it to a coworker who had helped me move out of my house the night I moved to the homeless project. She asked me several times if I was sure I didn't want to sell it, and I was. My only condition was that she use it often.

I had finally ridden a bike in Florida, and that same bike would become my transportation for months to come. Using a bungee cord, I would strap one of my collapsible canes to its frame and ride the bike wherever I needed to go. After a few months, I no longer needed to bring a cane along. I even taught my dogs to run alongside me as I rode, one at a time, of course. Amoré had the biggest smile ever as he loped long next to me and the bike, while Duke wanted to run on forever.

I was like a little kid, doing things that I never thought I would ever be able to do again. My level of appreciation for each "new" thing I was able to do was incredible. I don't think I had ever been happier and I would continue to get even happier as the months and years with the pump wore on.

I didn't have much trouble getting to sleep that night after going eight miles on a bike. It was a good tired, a weariness brought on by good old fashion exercise. Imagine that, I remember thinking, me riding a bike, the same me who not so long before was celebrating being able to hobble a few steps on Marilyn's patio, thinking that would probably be as close to walking as I would ever get.

The pump was a time capsule, gradually and magically beaming me back to a place I thought no longer existed.

28

The pump had been implanted in March, 2007, and by February, 2008, I was no longer using a cane or any assistive equipment. By midsummer that year, I was off all medications. The pump dose was doing a great job at managing my symptoms and I was so happy to have a totally clear brain. I only had intermittent pain from the spasticity in the winter months and would manage that with a low dose medication.

In the spring, I had started working weekends at the day center for Clearwater Intervention Project (CHIP), one of the places I did homeless outreach therapy when I worked as in homeless outreach. I rode my bike to and from work and loved being back with the homeless population. I was able to do so much more than run the day services while I was working there, and it was wonderful to be able to make a difference again with a population I felt passionately about. I was volunteering with Dunedin Doggie Rescue almost full time and had been since December, 2007. I loved helping save dogs and helping people find a connection with a dog like the one I had with my dogs.

By the summer of 2008, I was also able to drive again, but it was an achievement that didn't come easy.

I had been having dreams about driving since the fall of 2007, but each time I got into someone's car to try in real life to press on the gas pedal, I still couldn't. My right leg and foot still couldn't press down the gas pedal or brake without jerking about. I wasn't sure that I would ever really be able to, but the dreams persisted much like the walking dreams had years before. The only difference was that there was no waking in a panic from the driving dreams. I was driving my neighbor's car in various dream scenes now and again. So, I felt like I had to keep trying every couple of months to see if I could.

One day that summer, I tried to press on the gas pedal and I could do it with one smooth motion. I was so excited. My friend let me drive us to our destination about two miles away, so I had to concentrate. I was not comfortable at all behind the wheel because at this point, it had been almost exactly six years since I had driven a car. But I got us there and made it home again. Driving a car wasn't even on my list of things I missed anymore, and there was no denying the excitement that surged through me when I discovered I could do it. I think I told everyone I knew, which by then had become an impressive number since I had had so many new friends in my life.

I was proud of my ever-growing list of new friends, and my newfound willingness to venture out and meet people. The pump and the mobility it brought had broadened my social horizons tremendously.

Marilyn helped me see that I could branch out socially without sacrificing anything. I also realized that as someone who had lost everything once, I had nothing left to lose by going out into the world and giving what I had.

I loved the energy of Marilyn's space, so the timing for my prolonged house sitting there was perfect. I was doing new things for the first time since the pump. It was almost as if I was someone else living someone else's life. I don't think I could have made the progress I made toward creating a new life if I had done it in my own place. She had a neighbor named Jack who already had become my friend. He would hold what we called "pickin' parties" in his backyard where local musicians would come and play and sing around a camp fire. That's where my social network got a jumpstart.

I had developed a profile on an online dating site in the

summer of 2007, although once I started going out with Duke to hear my friend Jack's band play around town, I started meeting plenty of people on my own. Well, with Duke's help. Jack would drive us to cute little place called The Purple Moon to hear his band, so Duke and I went on dates.

There were some outings where Duke would insist we go up to random people, and in doing so, I would have to initiate a conversation. Duke led me to some great humans in those early days of being out and about. One guy Duke insisted I talk to was a practicing Buddhist and jazz musician named Ray, who was listening to music too at "The Purple Moon." He gave me a proper introduction to yoga and we started to go together to hear other local musicians play.

The founders of the dog rescue, KK and Cathy, introduced me to everyone they knew and through the rescue events, I met even more dog-loving folks who also became part of my world. I was meeting people so rapidly that I was struggling to keep up. That was certainly a brand new problem for me to manage, but a welcome one.

I had known that I could create my life how I wanted it, but hadn't really ever taken the opportunity seriously. When I moved to Florida, I managed to create the same life I had in West Virginia, safe but hardly creative. This time was different. I went with almost every new opportunity that presented itself to see where it might take me. I wasn't afraid at all for the first time in my life. I knew that the pump's effectiveness was likely time-limited and I was experiencing everything as if I was a small child seeing wonders for the first time.

And really, that was exactly my perspective. Everything was exciting to me. I enjoyed every single second of every single thing that I was doing. I had never ventured into any experience devoid of fear in my life. I had a yearning to experience as much as I possibly could and felt there was an urgency to do it now. I didn't want to sit around at some undetermined future date and wish I had. I never wanted to do that again if I could help it.

One of the first adventures I had not long after the pump

was implanted was a flight to Washington, D.C., to visit a friend, and it was nice not to need wheelchair assistance for boarding. We even took a road trip from D.C. to Pittsburgh, so I could spend some time with my brother who was working there at the time and taking night courses toward an MBA.

It turned out to be the best visit I ever had with him.

We talked about our childhoods and marveled at the differences in our perceptions of the events we shared. As we talked, I finally understood his point of view about so many things. I didn't want that visit to end ever and was so thankful it was possible. As an added bonus, my brother encouraged me to check into online teaching because some of his graduate courses were online.

It was a piece of advice that eventually led me to a teaching position in the psychology department of University of Phoenix. I completed the phone interview process, the training process and was teaching my first two courses under the tutelage of a mentor by the early fall. Teaching under the mentor was still considered part of the hiring process, so once that evaluation was completed, I was hired to teach as an adjunct faculty member. I found I really liked online teaching. I found that my writing skills made it possible to convey my personality to the students, which had been my initial reservation about trying it.

Soon after that, my brave new world found me back behind the wheel of a car again. The couple who ran the doggie rescue –KK and Cathy-- agreed to give me their 1997 Mazda 626 if I would pay them back for the transmission repairs it needed. They let me pay for the work a little at a time and then the car became mine. I still had no credit from the bankruptcy. Early in 2008, I would never have thought that I would be driving and certainly never dreamed I would have a car before the year was out. It was as if I was living in someone else's dream. Almost as if the scars of the trauma of my life since 2003 were erased from my memory.

My 38th birthday in December of 2008 was the perfect combination of everything I loved. It fell on a Sunday and that Sunday happened to be a Suds on Sunday day. Suds on Sunday was a doggie rescue fundraiser held the first Sunday of each month and includes dog washing, dog adoptions, doggie items for sale, and live local musicians who volunteer their talents. Since it was December and too cold for a dog wash, we planned to have pictures with Santa for the dogs and dog owners. I had invited some clients from the homeless day center to come up and volunteer, and the only one who took me up of the invitation, a man named Dean, ended up playing Santa Claus after the Santa who was supposed to do it was a no-show.

    The Sunset Bridge Band, which included a few of my friends, supplied the entertainment. Someone brought me a pink crown, which I wore all day and my friends in the band made regular announcements that it was my birthday.

    Everyone kept wishing me a happy birthday. My boys had come earlier during set up to get their pictures taken with Santa and I was busy walking around to make sure things were being coordinated and going smoothly. I found myself stopping to really savor the day. I was standing at the far edge of the parking lot area, and I looked up at the porch at the Dunedin Brewery to see Santa taking a smoke break. Not far from where I was were the dog pens with the adoptable dogs, who barked and wagged their approval. There were people everywhere holding a beer in one hand and their dogs on a leash in the other. Laughter and smiles were everywhere.

    There could not have been a better place for me to celebrate my birthday, and what had been a truly amazing year.

29

The year 2009 did nothing to slow me down. I kayaked more. I camped more. I climbed a tree. I took a road trip in an RV to North Carolina with my dogs and three friends. But for me, that year will always be remember as the year I started running again.

In August, I asked my pump doctors if I could try to learn to run again. They said sure, if it didn't hurt, do it. So, I decided to do it right and had a friend of mine I knew through the rescue properly train me. Her name was Suzanne, who not only was an outstanding distance runner and triathlete but coordinated many of the area's most popular races. She did an awesome job preparing me.

My first goal was to run a mile by the date of Sarah's Magnificent Mile event in September held in Raleigh, N.C., which is a research fundraiser for both my illness and Spastic Paraplegia Foundation. I couldn't make it to Raleigh, so we did a little fundraiser here and a one mile run for Sarah. Sarah, who is the only person my age with PLS that I had met in the online PLS forums, had done this fundraiser for a couple of years and each year it had gotten bigger and better. Sarah and I continued to keep in touch.

Suzanne started me out with good warm ups and running only in short intervals. After a couple of weeks of that, we were doing longer intervals and some intermittent sprints. The sprints were amazing. I had forgotten about sprinting, but my body hadn't forgotten. I was still fast. Suzanne kept marveling that I looked like a gazelle when I sprinted.

I felt like I was unleashed, unencumbered and was amazed that I could do this again. My smile doesn't get any wider than it did that first sprint. I had run the equivalent of a mile once before the Magnificent Mile date. The week before the race day, I had a horrible chest cold and was having trouble breathing. I wasn't sure how the running would go on what would be a humid, sunny mid-September day.

Dawn and Rick, a couple friends I had met through the doggie rescue, ran with me and a few others on the mile course that Suzi set up for us at Hammock Park in Dunedin. Others came to cheer us on. Dawn and I made Rick watch "Fried Green Tomatoes" a night or two before the race, so during the race we all yelled, "Tawanda!"

Suzanne ran with me and my goal was to run it in 10 minutes. It was a rough mile for my congested lungs, but Suzanne kept me going and helped me regulate my breathing. I met my goal of 10 minutes and it was awesome. I made us some tags the day of the race to safety pin to our shirts when we ran our mile that said "4 Sarah." We took pictures to send to Sarah. Even the people who didn't run with us, but served as our cheerleaders, pitched in some money to send in for the "part-fundraiser, part-holy crap Tawny is actually running again" event.

Everyone knew about Sarah at this point. This was one of those moments that certainly was richer for being able to share it with friends. I would run another one mile race early in October and we finished that one in under nine minutes.

I continued to run in 2010, doing my first 5K, part of busy weekend of road races during Gasparilla in February. I followed that up a month later by running a popular Dunedin 5K called The Hog Hustle, and completed a third 5K in The Midnight Run along the Dunedin Causeway on July Fourth weekend.

Early in 2010, I decided it was time to let go of all the responsibility I had taken on with the doggie rescue. It was a sad and difficult thing for me to do. I wasn't great at letting go, but knew that it was time to let new and fresh enter. I resigned as vice president of the volunteer group, but continued to emcee at dog washes and helping out where I could.

Next I turned my attention to my Duke. I wanted to find him

a job since his role as my protector and overseer had all but vanished with the mobility the pump had given me. He seemed to enjoy being the one to help me when I wasn't stable, but he hadn't had any real work in quite some time. I decided to get him certified as a therapy dog. I wasn't sure where I wanted to go with him to work, but knew wherever we ended up, would be where we were needed.

30

With his new royal blue leash and matching collar, Duke seemed to share my excitement as I was getting us ready to leave to take him to work on his first day at the Homeless Emergency Project (HEP). Amore got a peanut butter and treat filled Kong toy right before Duke and I snuck out the back door to the car. Duke had his leash in his mouth and was prancing through the yard to the gate, tail and butt wagging wildly.

As we pulled into the HEP campus, which had grown considerably in my nearly five-year absence, I decided to park in the visitor parking in the lot off the main office. Much of this part of the campus was newer. Duke was barking his high-pitched excited bark as we parked and came barreling out of the backseat when I opened the door and grabbed his leash.

I found myself taking several deep breaths as I let him do some sniffing around the bushes around the parking lot. I was excited, yes, but I realized that I was also very anxious. My heart was racing as I looked around and saw familiar sites. Emotions flooded back from years ago that I thought had been erased. Flashes of memories from time spent in the dental clinic hit me as Duke pulled me around the next set of bushes by the entrance of the clinic.

That flash of memories led to more flashes of memories. I had a knot in the pit of my stomach from this rush of memories and emotions. I didn't realize I had underestimated the level of trauma I had experienced by the illness/homelessness experience, but my body was reminding me.

I took more deep breaths, reminding myself that I was ok now. I was living a different life than before and now we were here to give back—Duke and I together. With a final deep breath and a tug and "let's go" to Duke, we started walking into the main offices to then figure out where to go next. Familiar faces were mixed with unfamiliar faces and names. Familiar faces came with hugs and warm welcomes as many of the same people who were there when I both worked and lived at HEP were still there. I introduced Duke to everyone and he was eating up the attention.

The volunteer coordinator took us around to introduce us to residents and for a tour of the newer buildings and programs. We were warmly received by everyone we encountered, and I worried Duke might throw out a hip from all of his wagging.

I was a bit disoriented at times during the tour. My most recent memories of being there were all from a seated position in a wheelchair, so my memory of where buildings were in relationship to everything else was often wrong. I would have sworn the community center was located somewhere else and even joked that they must have moved the building.

The apartment building I lived in looked exactly the same, but there was a new apartment building on the asphalt parking lot facing it. Seeing it up close with Duke made my heart race and I started to sweat a bit. One of the staff suggested that I stop in to visit someone that lived in apartment #4, so Duke and I headed over there by ourselves to make introductions.

We first walked over to the estuary's edge to take a few deep breaths. Memories of ducks and herons and fishing poles were flitting through my mind. I told Duke quickly that this is where his mommy kept her sanity when she was away from him. He sniffed around quite a bit while I prepared myself to go up to apartment 4 to knock on the door.

I had forgotten that I lived in apartment 4 and without thinking, took Duke up the wheelchair ramp instead of the stairs to get to it. We introduced ourselves, briefly went inside the apartment to meet the client when Duke just let himself in the front door, and then went for a walk with the client around the campus. The apartment was arranged differently, but was essentially the same as I remembered it. I found it fitting that our first referral was to my old apartment. I hold both fond and frightening memories of my time there and all of them flashed into my mind almost as if it was one single event in time, rather than many memories over a six month period.

Duke and I explored the terrain that I made that power wheel chair traverse during my stay there. I have no idea how I made it go out there by the water or behind the apartment building. Duke was getting hot with all of the walking around in the sun, and it was time for us to leave, so we headed back toward the main office to the car.

Every place I looked seemed to hold some significance in my mind that lead to a surge of emotions and memories, so I was pretty tired as I tried to process the day in my mind on the way back to the car from the apartments.

We were there to give back and it seemed everyone was on board to help us do just that. It was exciting to be there with one of my dogs to do it with me, but I hadn't expected the intensity of emotion being there would evoke. It must be time to process all of that now that I am back with my dogs, safe, and happier than I have ever been in my life. While the goal was giving back, I am not sure that both Duke and I won't benefit from the adventures and times that await us at HEP.

Duke became an official therapy dog through Project PUP (Pets Uplifting People) on May 8, 2010. Since I couldn't have my dogs when I lived at HEP, it seemed that being able to take Duke there might just help a lot of people the same way that Wayne's Sammy had helped me when I lived there. I also wasn't sure I wanted to go to a nursing home regularly, which is where most therapy dogs go—I wasn't ready to do that.

I didn't realize that I wasn't all that emotionally prepared to return to HEP either, until I got there. I really had "forgotten" so much about my time there at that point, that even where different places were on campus seemed confusing for me. Nothing seemed to be where I seemed to remember it was.

     Before we knew it, the demand for us in the different homeless programs had become overwhelming. We would spend more than the once a month the certifying organization had required, and instead we went once a week. Duke was phenomenal at this therapy dog stuff. I knew he was intuitive with me, but he would never cease to amaze me with different clients and staff on any given day we would go. He loved going so much that just getting his bandana on him was hard sometimes. He hadn't waggled like that ever that I could ever recall. He was happy and wonderful at his job. Soon, once a week turned into twice a week by the end of the year. As we celebrated our four-year anniversary and Duke's 13th birthday in May of 2014, we were seeing HEP residents three times a week as independent contractors.

     On that first day, some staff and residents were in the parking lot as I was opening the back door to let Duke jump in, so we said our good-byes as I got in behind the wheel. What a great time Duke and I had together today, and what an emotional rollercoaster trip down memory lane. In my days of sitting by the estuary in my wheelchair, fighting off the darkness, feeding the ducks, dealing with my pain, I never could have dreamed of a day as wonderful as today.

     As I waved and pulled out of the parking lot, I realized there would be no bargaining with God to get me safely home. Now, I would only be thanking him.

Epilogue

    I was able to get the book written, but not published, before losing my boys to old age. Duke was able to serve at HEP for five years before he died at the age of 14—plaques memorialize him in two spots on campus. His brother preceded him in death at age 13.

    As Duke was slowing down, I had an opportunity to go to Stanford University to become a Master Trainer in the Chronic Disease Self-Management program and bring that program to HEP. I am currently Wellness Program Manager at HEP's Dental and Wellness Clinic, and in 2016 was named one of the Tampa Bay Lightning's Community Heroes for my service at HEP. I also serve as volunteer Secretary of the Board of Directors for Project PUP—Pets Uplifting People, and continue in my role as adjunct faculty for University of Phoenix.

    My newest rescue Hope Fiona and I still live in Dunedin, FL.

Acknowledgements

    This book took a village and each contribution is deeply appreciated. I cannot possibly name everyone of my family and my friends near and far, but I do want to specifically thank Jen Cybulski for sharing her talent on the cover and Dan Howley for his ability to pare down so much material from the original manuscript. Rebecca Lett stepped up at the end to finalize the back cover and spine. There hasn't been a human on my path who hasn't supported the creation and publication of this story.
    I would be remiss not to mention my family at the Homeless Empowerment Program (HEP) and it was actually the impetus for finally getting this book out there to you. It became a project to give back to them, so 20% of any monies generated from the sale of this book will go to the Dental and Wellness Clinic at HEP.